# Velveteen Rabbit's

## Life Lessons

# Velveteen Rabbit's

## Life Lessons

Harriet Griffey

*Illustrated by* Emma Carlisle

RIZZOLI
UNIVERSE

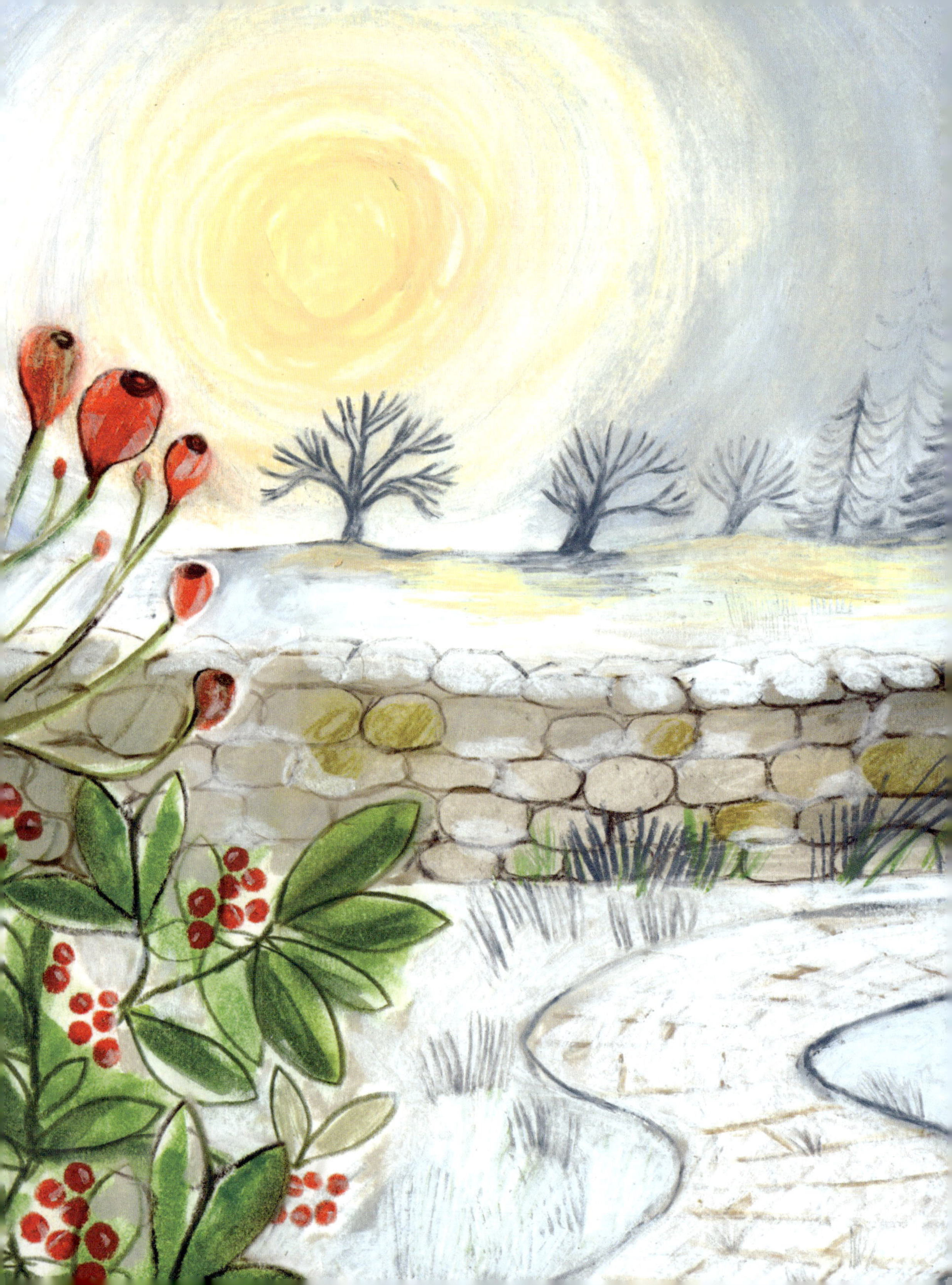

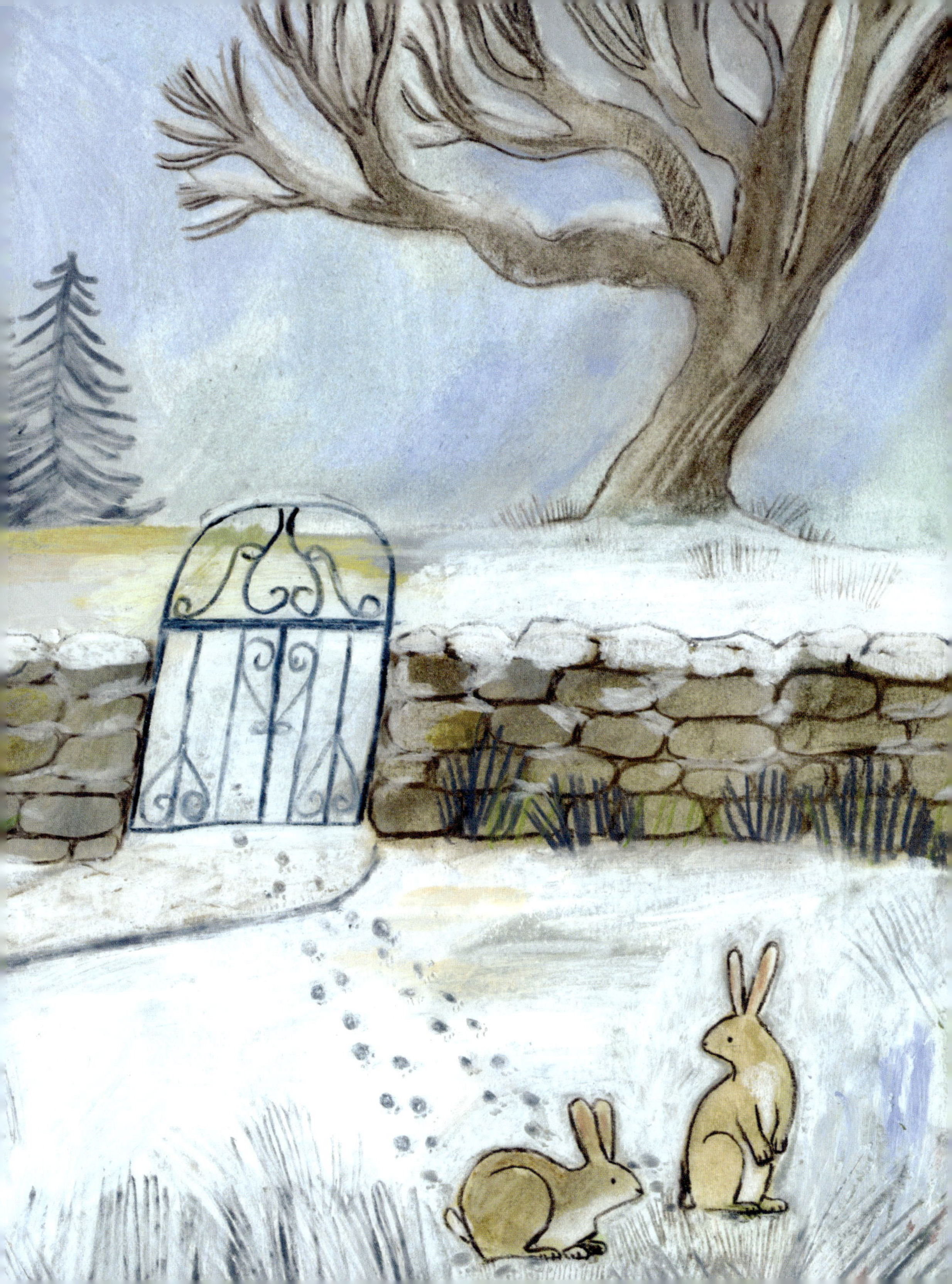

# Introduction

The beloved children's book *The Velveteen Rabbit (or, How Toys Become Real)* is the story of a child's love for his toy rabbit and how, through this love, the rabbit becomes real.

Published in 1922, the same year as T. S. Eliot's *The Waste Land*, F. Scott Fitzgerald's *The Great Gatsby*, and James Joyce's *Ulysses*, *The Velveteen Rabbit* is among the great literary works of its day. Four years after the devastation of World War I, its author Margery Williams recognized that a bruised and battered world needed words of consolation.

Given to a young boy as a Christmas present, the Velveteen Rabbit at first feels overlooked among showier toys. He learns from the wise old Skin Horse that toys become real when they are truly loved by a child. The Rabbit eventually becomes the boy's favorite companion, and through their deep bond he feels real in a heartfelt, emotional sense. When the boy falls ill with scarlet fever, the Rabbit stays by his side. After the boy recovers, however, the doctor orders all contaminated toys to be burned—including the Rabbit. Heartbroken, the Velveteen Rabbit is left outside, where a Nursery Magic Fairy appears. Because of the boy's genuine love, she transforms the toy into a real, living rabbit. The complete story can be read at the end of this book (see pages 90–95).

Readers young and old have long recognized the universal truths enshrined in Williams' text—the importance of authenticity, the value of resilience, that true happiness comes from self-acceptance, it's OK to feel sad, good relationships take work, and love lies at the heart of everything.

This new book distills these core truths from the original text and, alongside contemporary and inspirational commentary, reflects the wisdom of *The Velveteen Rabbit* for a whole new generation of readers.

*There was once a velveteen rabbit, and in the beginning he was really splendid.*

At every child's birth, there is a promise of amazing possibilities and potential. These are realized through the daily living of life's many lessons.

Sometimes those lessons are hard, and we can feel that life is unfair or too difficult, but often those lessons are delightful, and we can learn from moments of fun, awe, and inspiration too. The flourishing of one's true self is a genuinely positive aim.

Remaining optimistic when negative things happen can be tough, but it's important to store up positive experiences and look for the beauty in the world each and every day.

*A happy life starts with a*
*promise to yourself to seek it.*

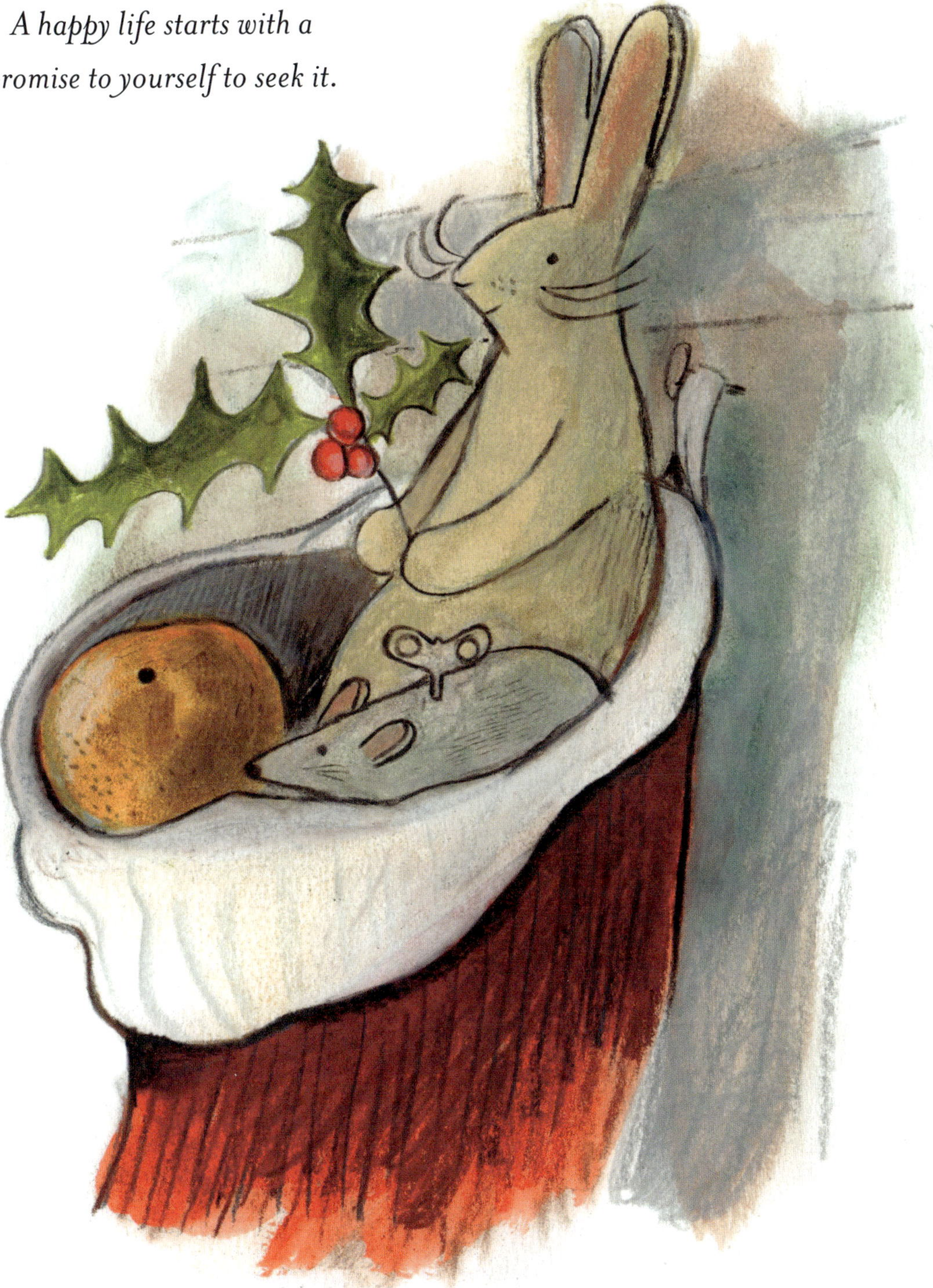

On Christmas morning, when he sat wedged in the top of the Boy's stocking, with a spring of holly between his paws, the effect was charming ... For at least two hours the Boy loved him, and then ... in the excitement of looking at all the new presents the Velveteen Rabbit was forgotten.

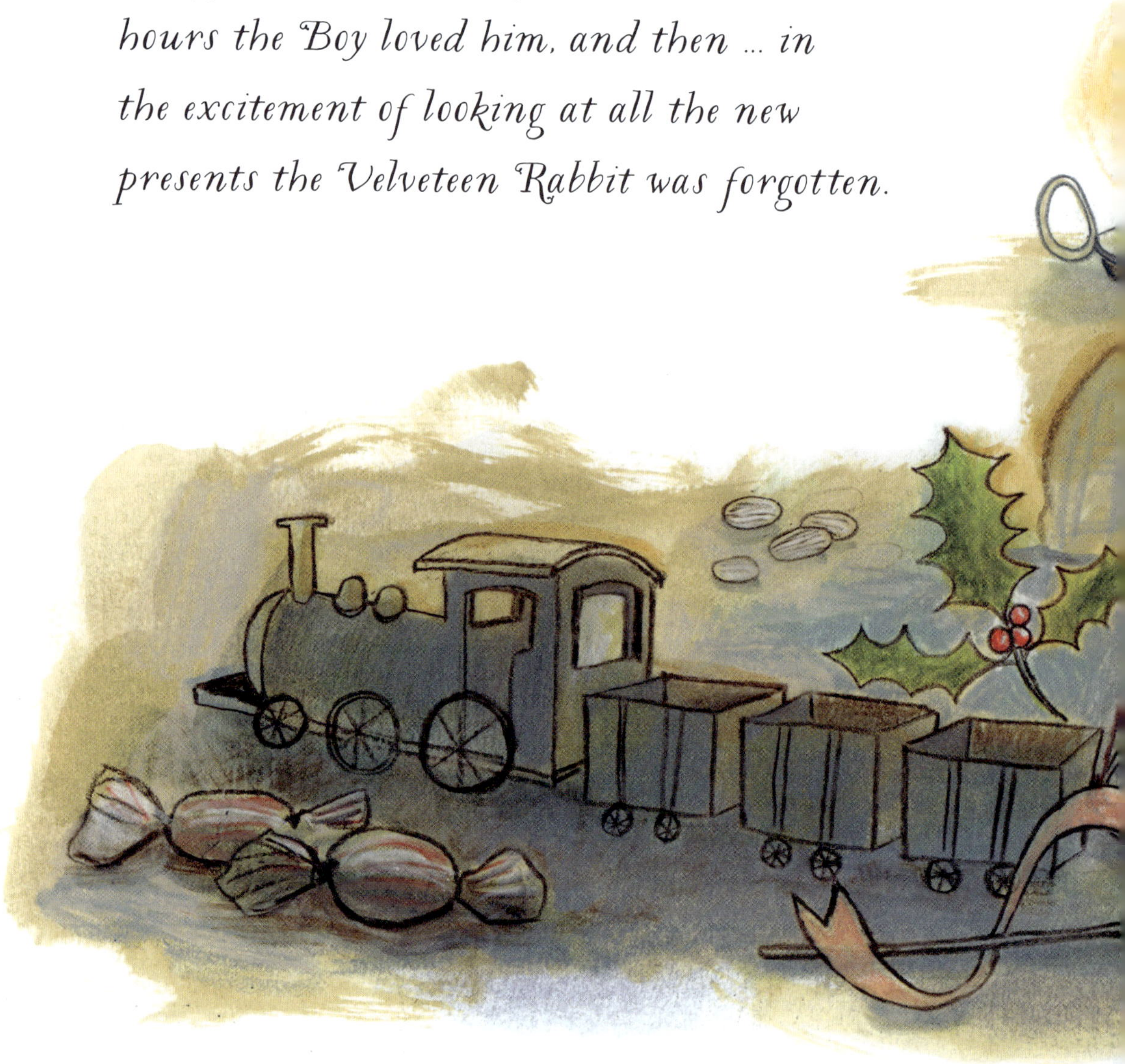

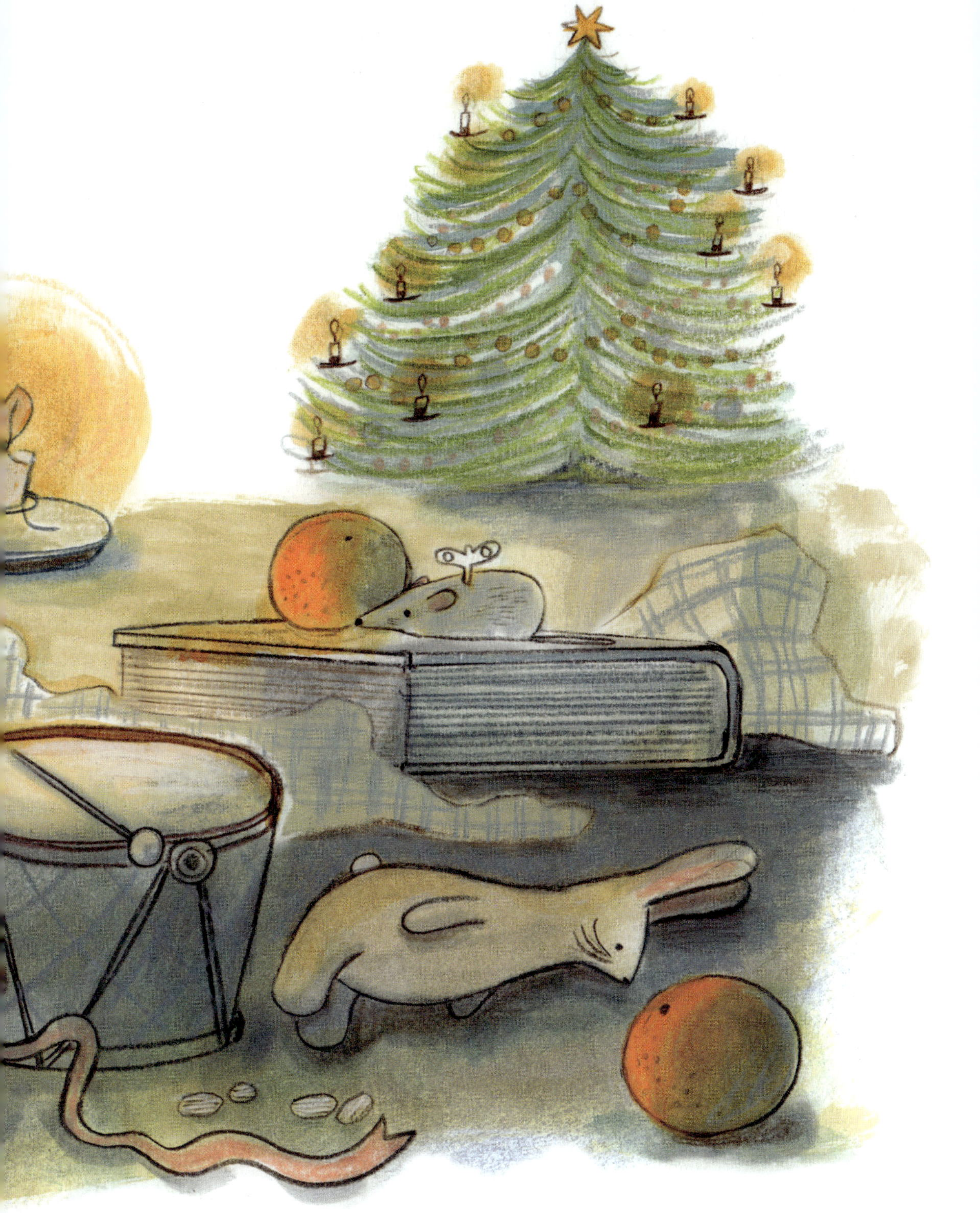

One of life's many lessons is that things never remain the same. Circumstances, situations, and even people can change. Whether this is good or bad depends on how we see things or view change. Some of us embrace it while some of us are more cautious, but accepting and accommodating change is part of how we grow.

Alongside moments of happiness and joy can be those of difficulty and sadness, when we might feel despondent, forgotten, or inconsequential. But there are always choices to be made about how we respond to what happens, and this gives us agency and control over how we feel.

*Don't base your happiness on things outside your control, but on those things that you can control, like your thoughts, actions, and mindset.*

*For a long time he lived in the toy cupboard or on the nursery floor, and no one thought very much about him. He was naturally shy, and being only made of velveteen, some of the more expensive toys quite snubbed him.*

All relationships teach us something, even when others are sometimes thoughtless or unkind.

It's not just what happens to us, but how we respond to it that is important. It can help to recognize that you always have a choice about how you wish to respond and exercising that choice will help you retain your power.

*Your worth isn't determined by how others see or treat you—and growth often happens quietly, without recognition.*

*The mechanical toys were very superior,
and looked down upon everyone else;
they were full of modern ideas, and
pretended they were Real.*

Not everyone will share your values, but it doesn't mean you should discard them in order to fit in. First and foremost, being true to yourself is what matters.

We all travel through life with our own ideas and emotional baggage; the trick is to find those points of similarity between ourselves and others, rather than focus on any differences. Accepting someone else's right to their own point of view, even while you may not agree with it, is the basis of a civilized society.

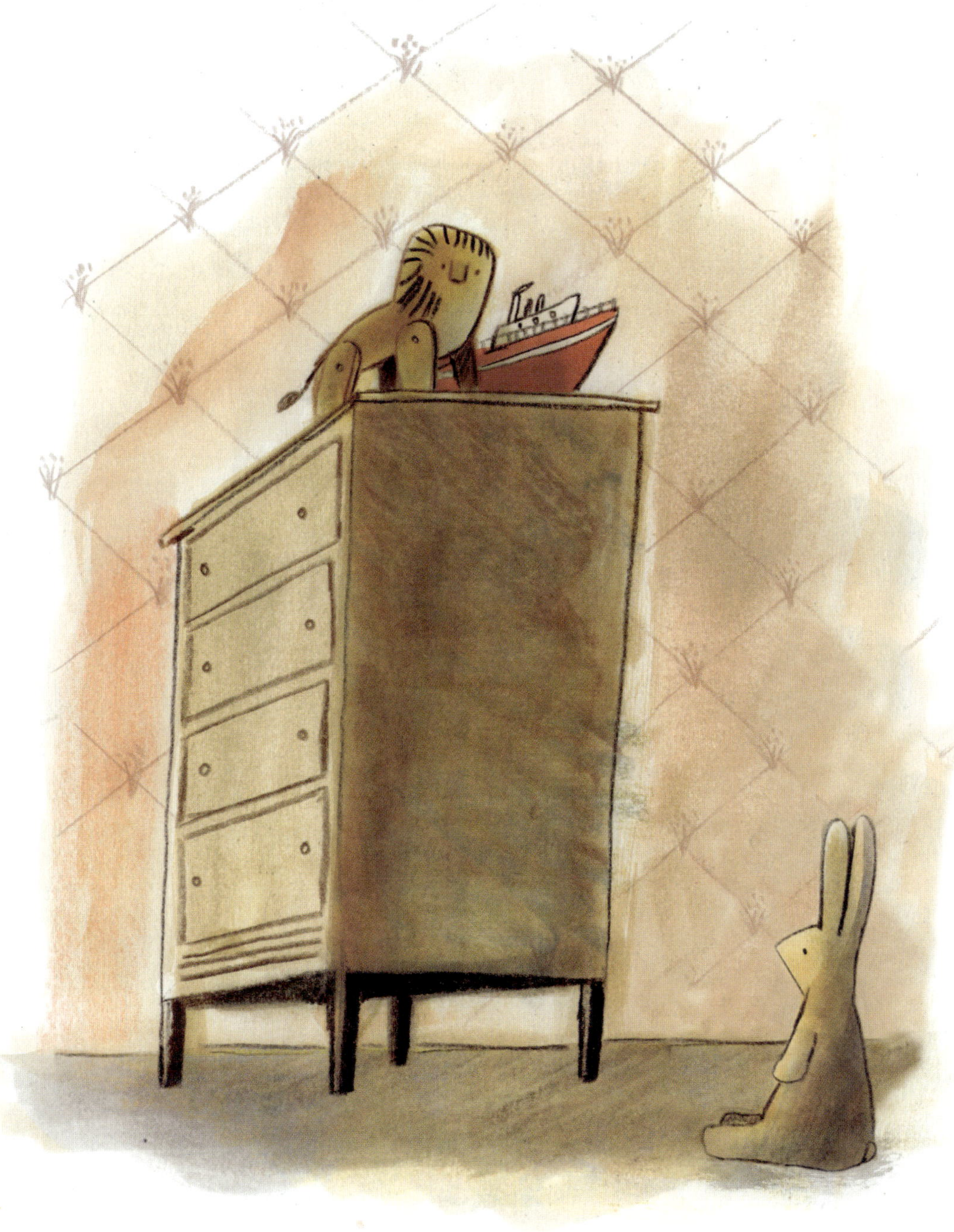

*Being authentic to your own self gives you the power to make the choices that are right for you.*

*Between them all the poor little Rabbit was made to feel himself very insignificant and commonplace, and the only person who was kind to him at all was the Skin Horse.*

Do not give other people the power to make you feel small and insignificant.

Their opinion of you may be based on prejudice or lack of knowledge and it is only the opinion of those who know and love us that should carry any real weight or value.

Not everyone will share your aims and dreams, so look for connections to those who treat you with the same consideration and kindness that you offer to them.

*If someone seeks to undermine you or diminish your power, that's their weakness not yours.*

*The Skin Horse had lived longer in the nursery than any of the others. He was so old that his brown coat was bald in patches ... He was wise.*

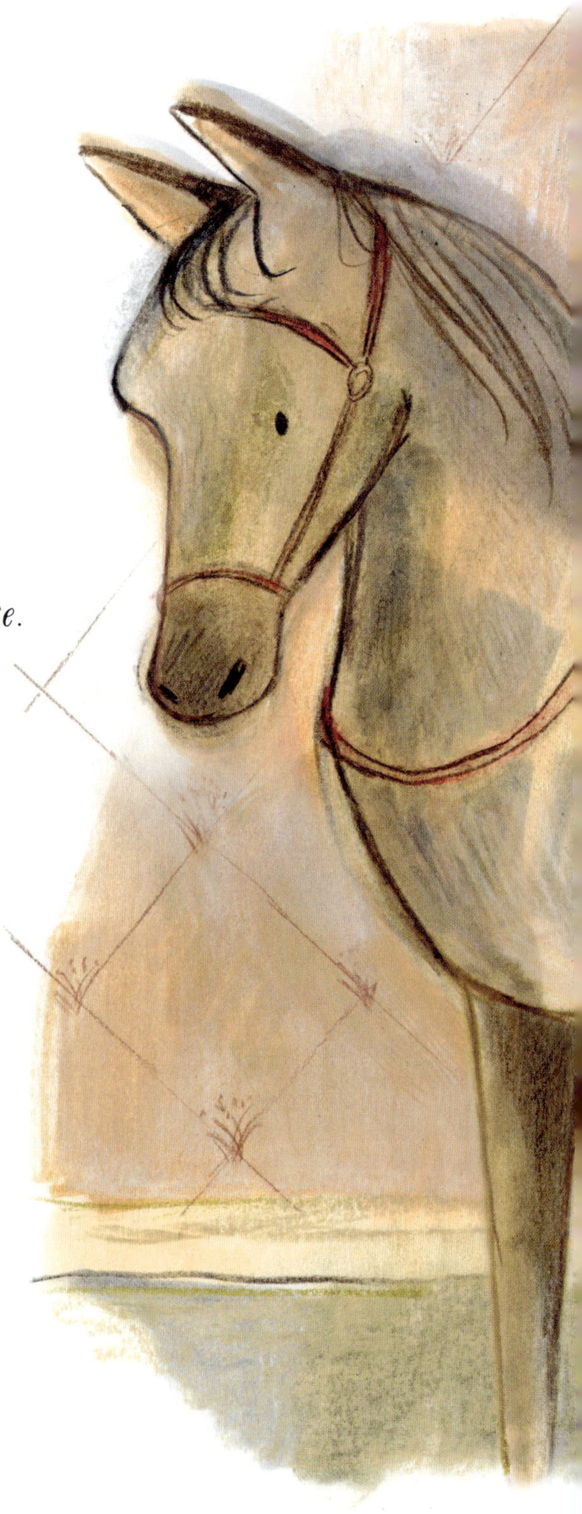

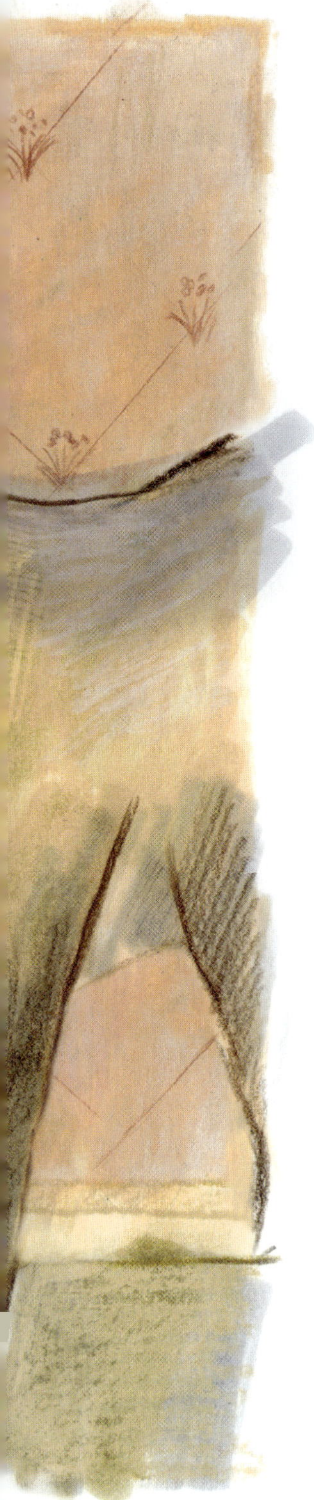

What is wisdom?

Wisdom involves making decisions based on experience and knowledge and applying insights gained over time. It also involves an ability to reflect on human nature—our own and other people's—which is often subject to change, contradiction, and uncertainty.

Age isn't a requirement for wisdom, but the ability to reflect on life's experiences without judgement is something that takes practice and time. Often, it's through listening to and sharing in the experiences of others that we can gain perspective—perspective that helps us to respond to life with authenticity and wisdom.

*One day, looking back with hard-won wisdom,*
*everything will make perfect sense.*

*"What is REAL?" asked the Rabbit one day ...*
*"Real isn't how you are made," said the Skin Horse.*
*"It's a thing that happens to you. When a child loves you for a long, long time, not just to play with, but REALLY loves you, then you become Real."*

Being real, being true to ourselves and our personal values, is sometimes hard in today's world but it's important to have our own personal compass on which to rely.

Being real comes from developing a strong sense of self, and this self-realization of who we are and what we value and believe in, will be invaluable in providing a polestar for the life decisions we need to make.

Authenticity isn't always the easy option, but it will sit more comfortably over time as we learn to trust the wisdom of staying true to ourselves.

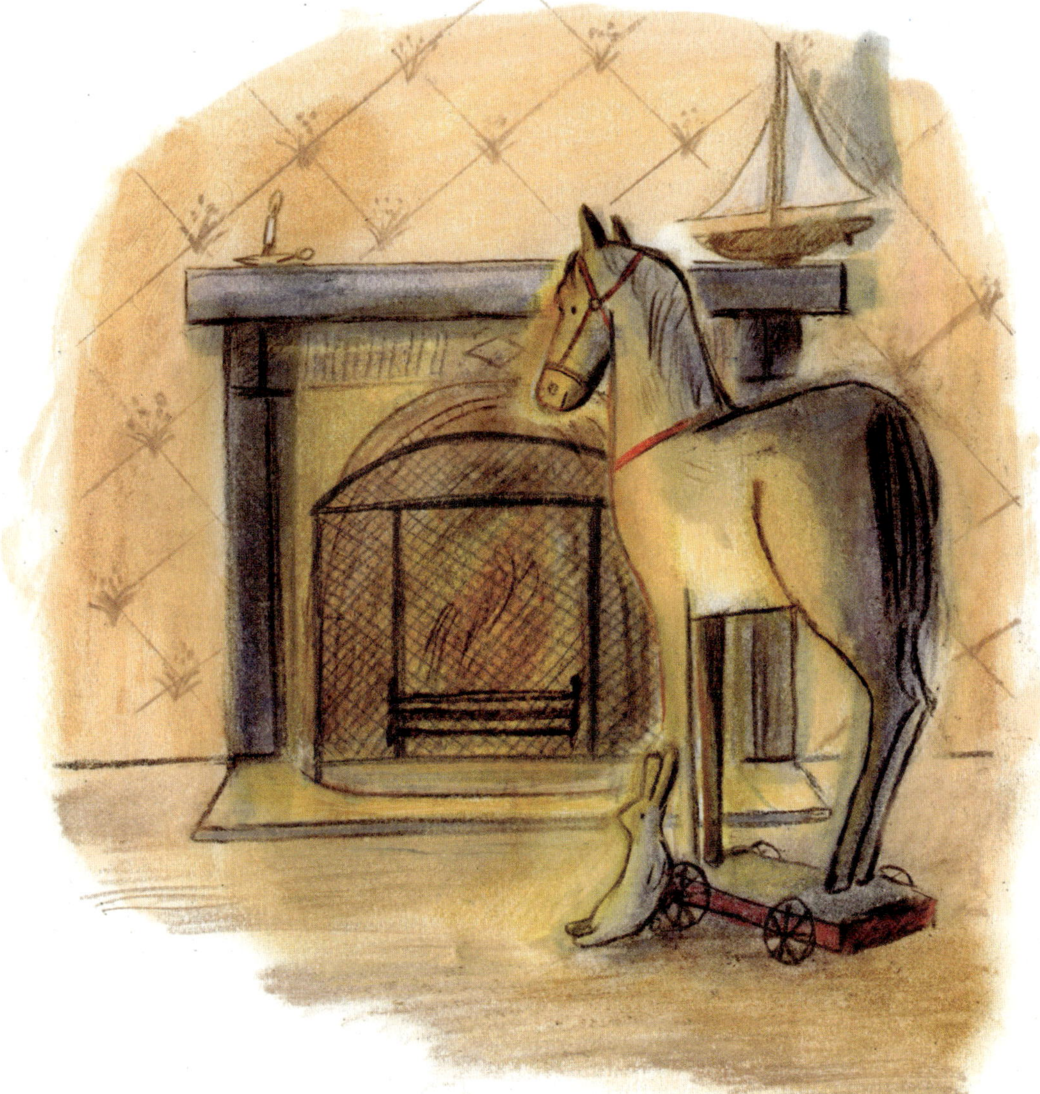

*If we choose relationships with those whose values align with our own, it makes it easier to stay true to what matters to us.*

*"Does it hurt?" asked the Rabbit.*

*"Sometimes," said the Skin Horse, for he was always truthful. "When you are Real you don't mind being hurt."*

Emotional pain teaches us that we have feelings and that these feelings matter.

We can feel hurt by loss, grief, despair, loneliness, and other human experience, and these feelings are an appropriate response to pain. When someone we love dies, for example, feeling sad is a normal response. It hurts, but we learn to manage the sadness of it.

Emotions can sometimes be difficult to identify and manage, and we can feel overwhelmed by them. But if we reflect on how we feel, this will deepen our understanding of our feelings. Self-awareness can be supported by developing good relationships with those we trust and on whom we can rely when times are tricky.

*Grief is a response to loss that can take time and acceptance to process. Be as gentle on yourself as you would be with others.*

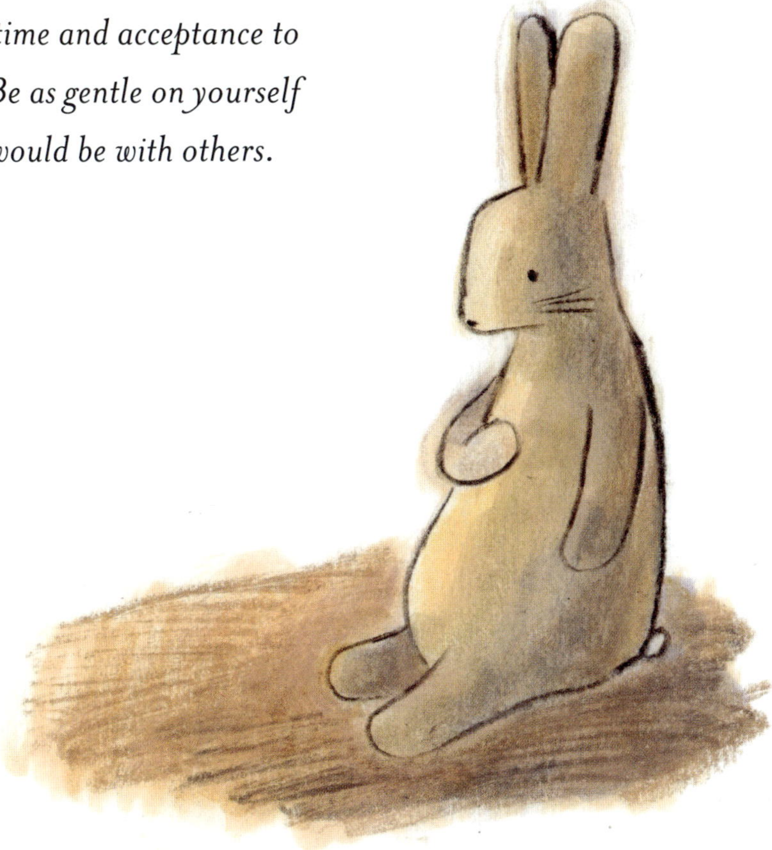

*"Does it happen all at once ..." he asked, "or bit by bit?"*

*"It doesn't happen all at once," said the Skin Horse. "You become. It takes a long time ... by the time you are Real, most of your hair has been loved off, and your eyes drop out and you get loose in the joints and very shabby. But these things don't matter at all, because once you are Real you can't be ugly, except to people who don't understand."*

Judging someone on their looks is a superficial response, but a very common way in which to form initial impressions about someone. We all do it, so it's good to be aware of the potential for prejudice and to remind ourselves that we wouldn't want to be judged in this superficial way.

Self-acceptance of our own strengths and weaknesses can help us accept those of others too, but that degree of self-awareness takes time and life experience to develop. Aging can affect us physically, but as long as we stay open minded and curious, we stay beautiful.

*Becoming real is empowering; learning to trust how we feel and responding with authenticity is key.*

*"I suppose you are Real?" said the Rabbit. And then he wished he had not said it, for he thought the Skin Horse might be sensitive. But the Skin Horse only smiled ... "Once you are Real you can't become unreal again."*

Like a lot of life experience, it can take time for feelings of authenticity to become embedded in the way we respond and react. From this, a genuine sense of self-confidence can grow.

Few of us are naturally and immediately self-confident. It can be helpful to remember that others often feel unsure in many situations too, even if their uncertainty isn't visible to us.

Asking questions like the little Rabbit, and listening to the answers, helps develop communication skills that encourage empathy. This, in turn, will also help us to respond with curiosity and kindness.

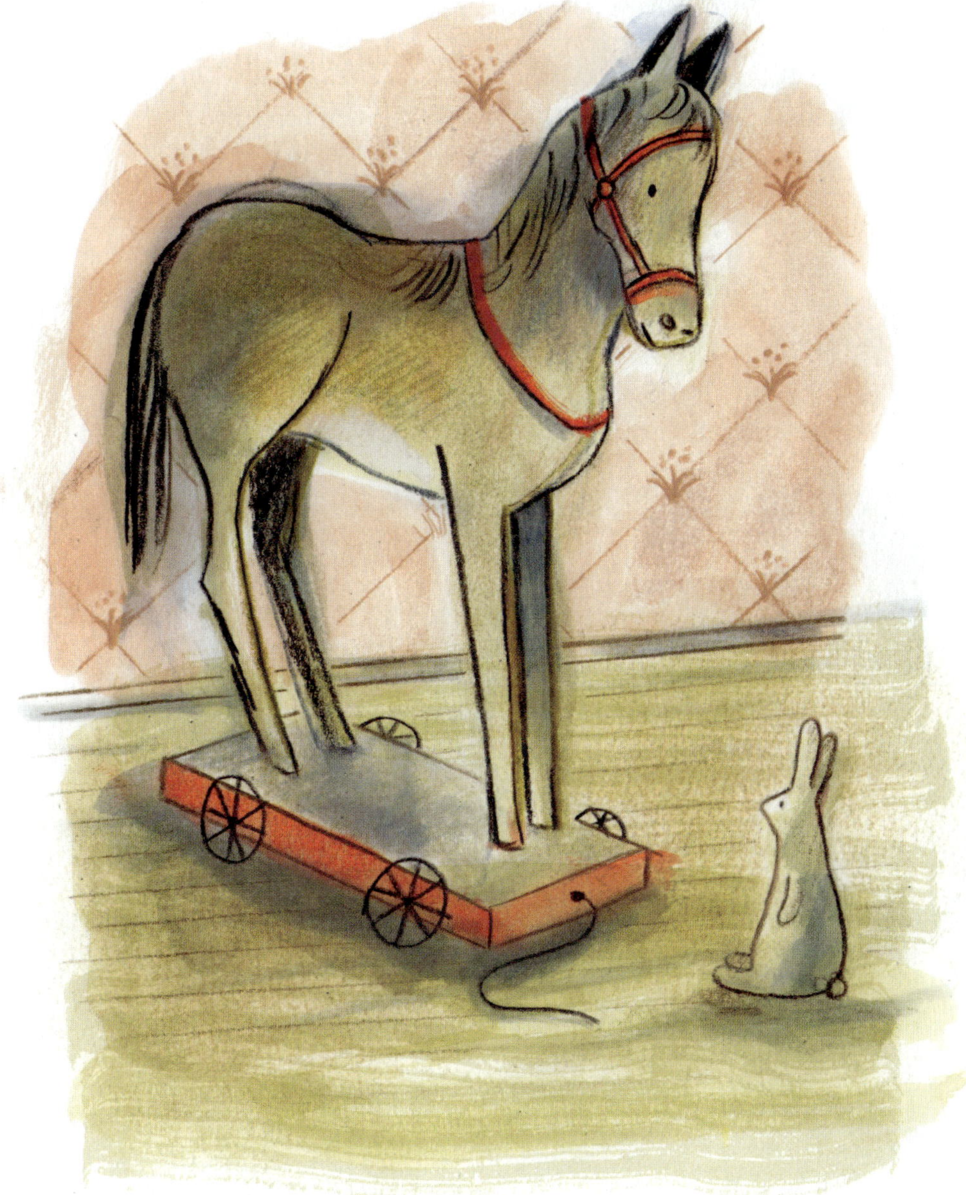

*Finding ways to put others at ease often helps us to feel more comfortable too.*

*The Rabbit sighed. He thought it would be a long time before this magic called Real happened to him. He longed to become Real, to know what it felt like; and yet the idea of growing shabby and losing his eyes and whiskers was rather sad.*

Magic is a name we sometimes give to something powerful, for which we often have no words.

Magic is also something we can make happen through our thoughts and actions, transforming ourselves by what we choose to believe and do. Thoughts become words, words become actions, actions become habits, and suddenly we have established and grounded ourselves in a new, positive reality.

We can't stop the passing of the years, and it is a privilege to have the time to realize our potential, so stay curious and open-minded about the magical world around you.

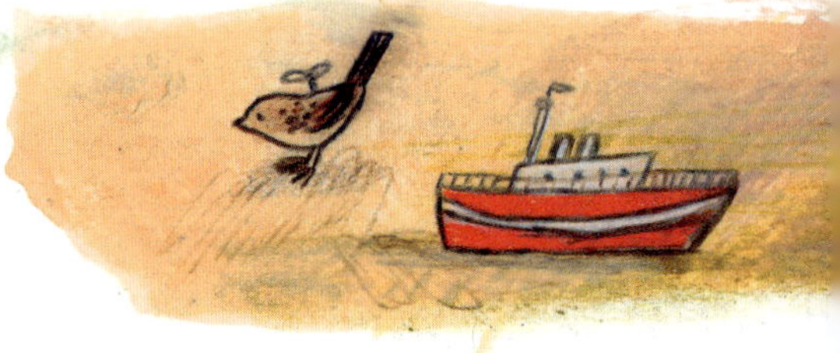

*Life isn't always easy, but there's always room for a little magic to enhance your day if you look for it.*

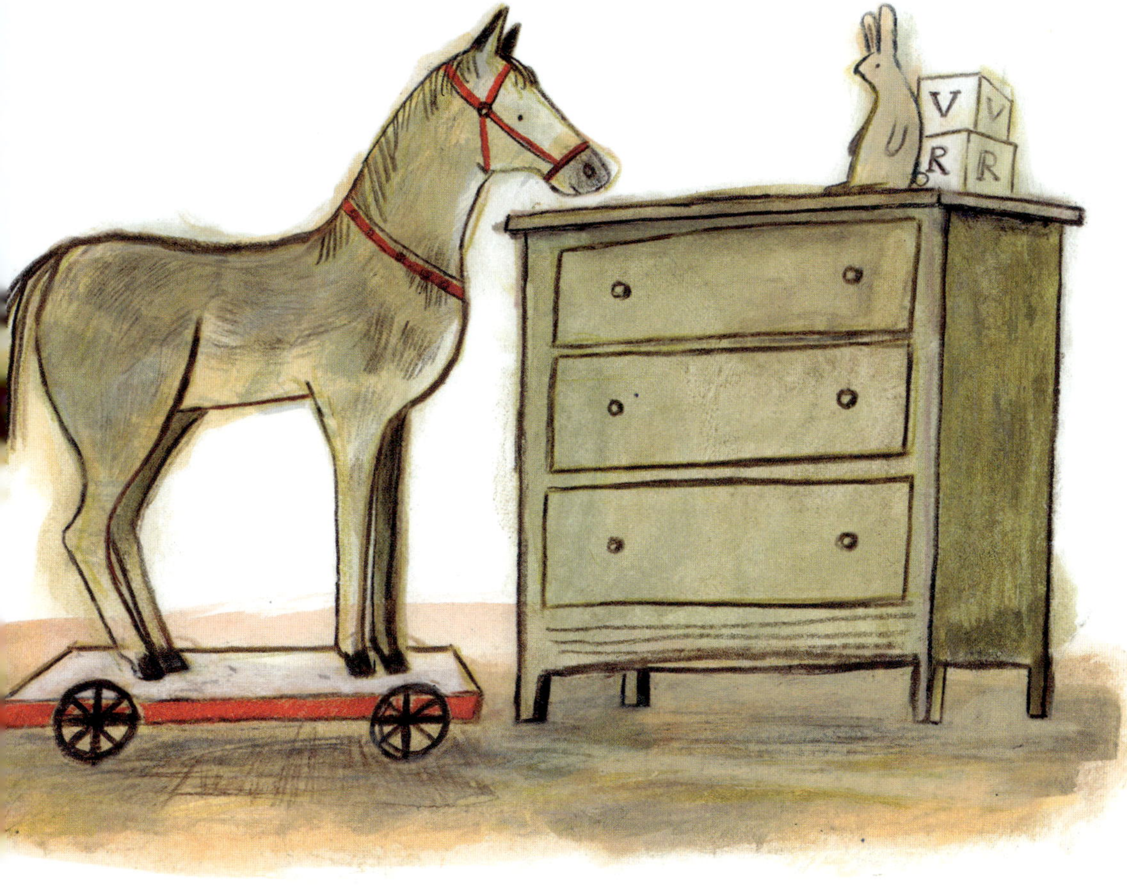

*One evening, when the Boy was going to bed, he couldn't find the china dog that always slept with him ... That night, and for many nights after, the Velveteen Rabbit slept in the Boy's bed ... And when the Boy dropped off to sleep, the Rabbit would snuggle down close.*

We can sometimes feel thrown by change, particularly when it puts us outside the reassurance of our comfort zone.

That's when it's good to remember that we are loved. As babies and infants, we are programed to seek out the love we need to grow emotionally and, as we grow, we internalize this experience of being loved. This, in turn, helps us feel secure and valued in the years to come, particularly when circumstances change or challenge us.

Love isn't finite—the more we love, the more love we have to give and receive. Keep your heart open to love but, at the same time, recognize where your love isn't valued and honored to protect your heart.

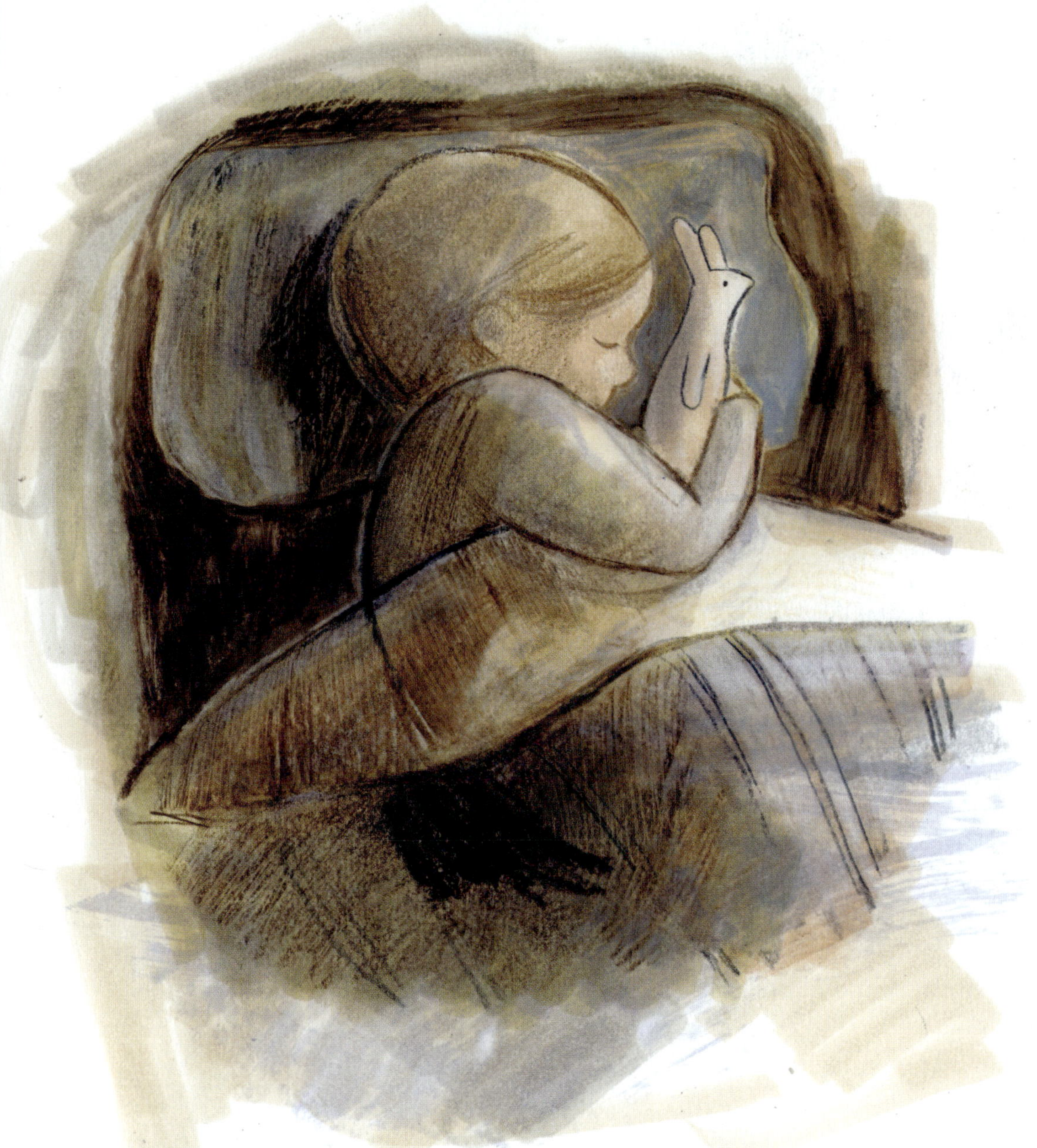

*A hug is a physical expression of love;*
*whenever you give one you receive one in return.*

*And so time went on, and the little Rabbit was very happy—so happy that he never noticed how his beautiful velveteen fur was getting shabbier and shabbier, and his tail becoming unsewn, and all the pink rubbed off his nose where the Boy had kissed him.*

Self-realization is a process where you come to know yourself, recognize your dreams, and fulfil your potential. This takes time and every life lesson helps you towards your own personal goal.

Rather than resist the passing of the years and hanging on to past negative experiences, actively look for new ideas and opportunities that will replenish your soul. Never stop looking and learning, as it is this that will keep you inspired.

*The past is not a place to live in, but to learn from.*

*Spring came, and they had long days in the garden, for wherever the Boy went the Rabbit went too … And once, the Rabbit was left out on the lawn until long after dusk, and Nana had to come and look for him … because the Boy couldn't go to sleep unless he was there … "Fancy all that fuss for a toy!" she said.*

Like the seasons, times change; so too, do circumstances, relationships, and our experience of life. Be open to these changes and remember that another person's difficulties may be a life lesson with which they are struggling; your patience with their struggle can be a gift to them.

Remember, too, that feelings always matter—our own and other people's. We may not have the exact same experiences on which to reflect or draw, but with curiosity and imagination it's always possible to see the world from another person's point of view.

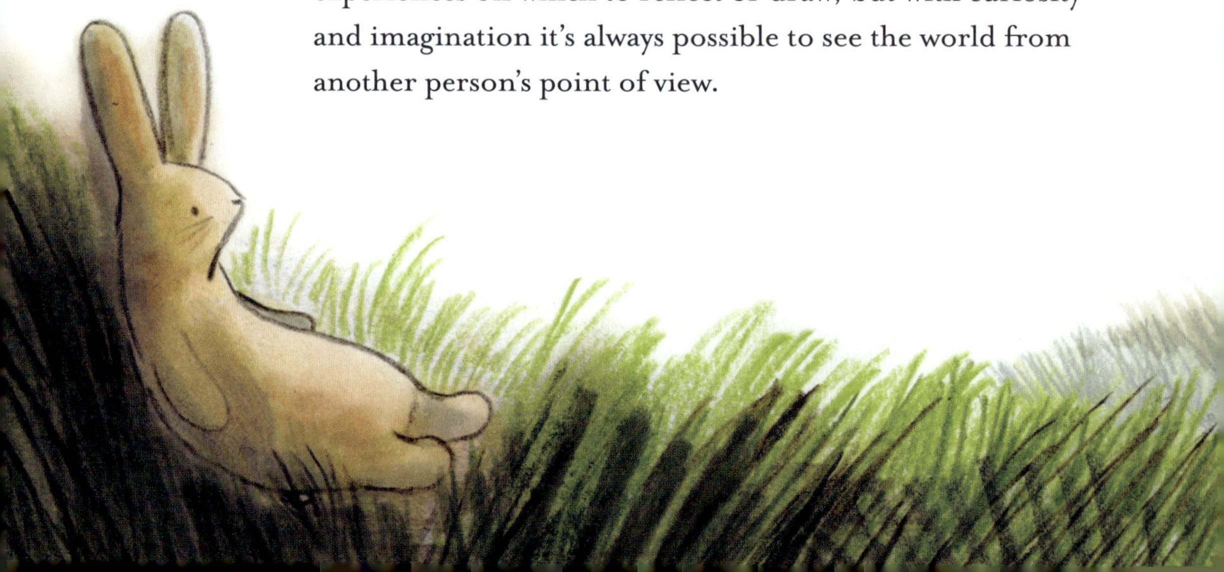

*Love is what gives something value, so be understanding to others. What may seem small or insignificant to you may mean everything to someone else.*

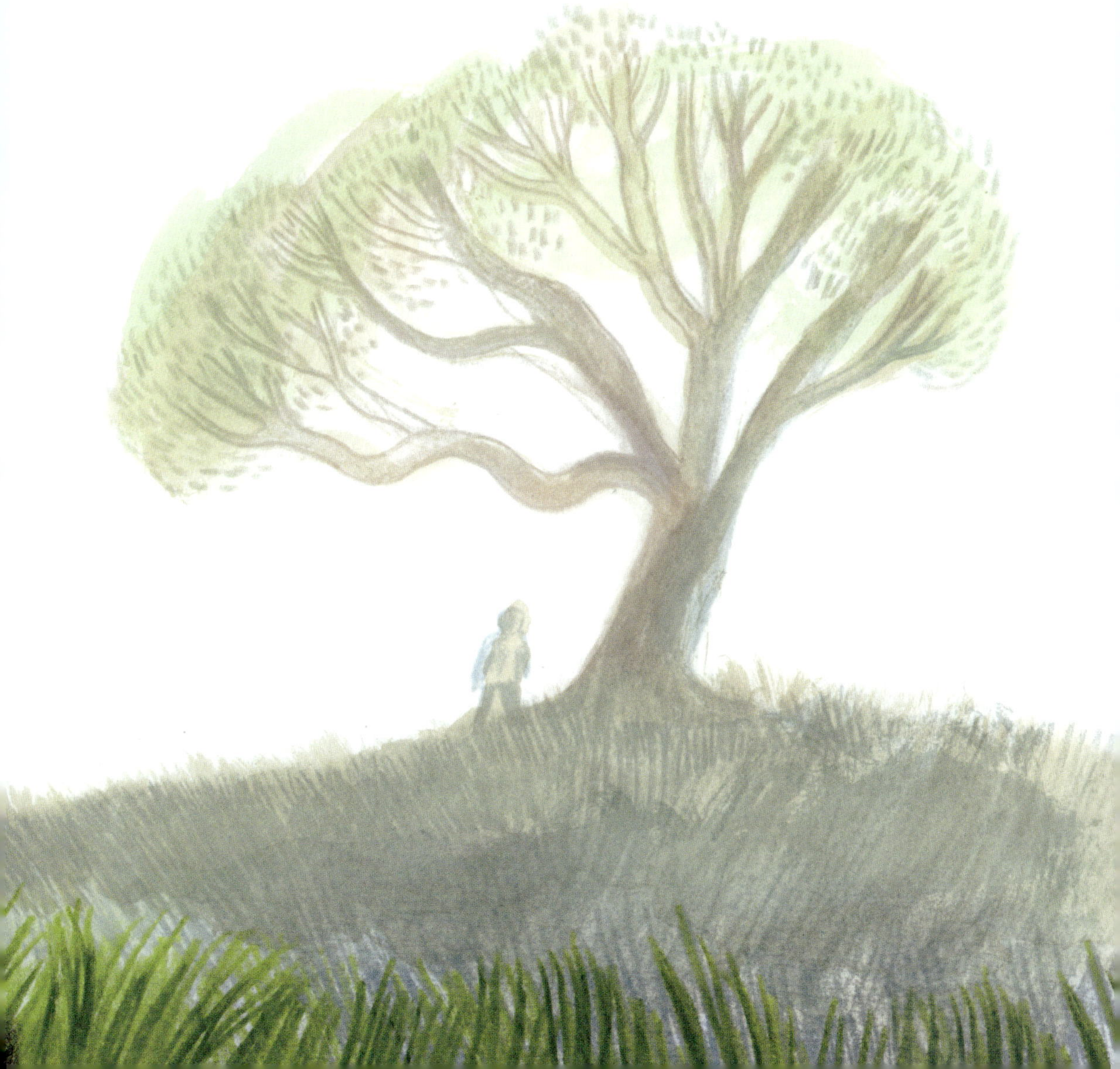

*The boy sat up in bed and stretched out his hands ... "You mustn't say that. He isn't a toy. He's REAL." When the little Rabbit heard that he was happy, for he knew that what the Skin Horse had said was true at last ... He was Real. The Boy himself had said it.*

Acknowledgment of how we feel helps build confidence in learning to manage and self-regulate our emotions.

Like the little Rabbit, having someone who values and cares about us, who believes in us, and acknowledges our attempts to manage how we feel, is hugely beneficial to our emotional wellbeing.

Likewise, do this for someone you care about too. Reciprocating love and care yields its own reward and helps nurture authentic relationships.

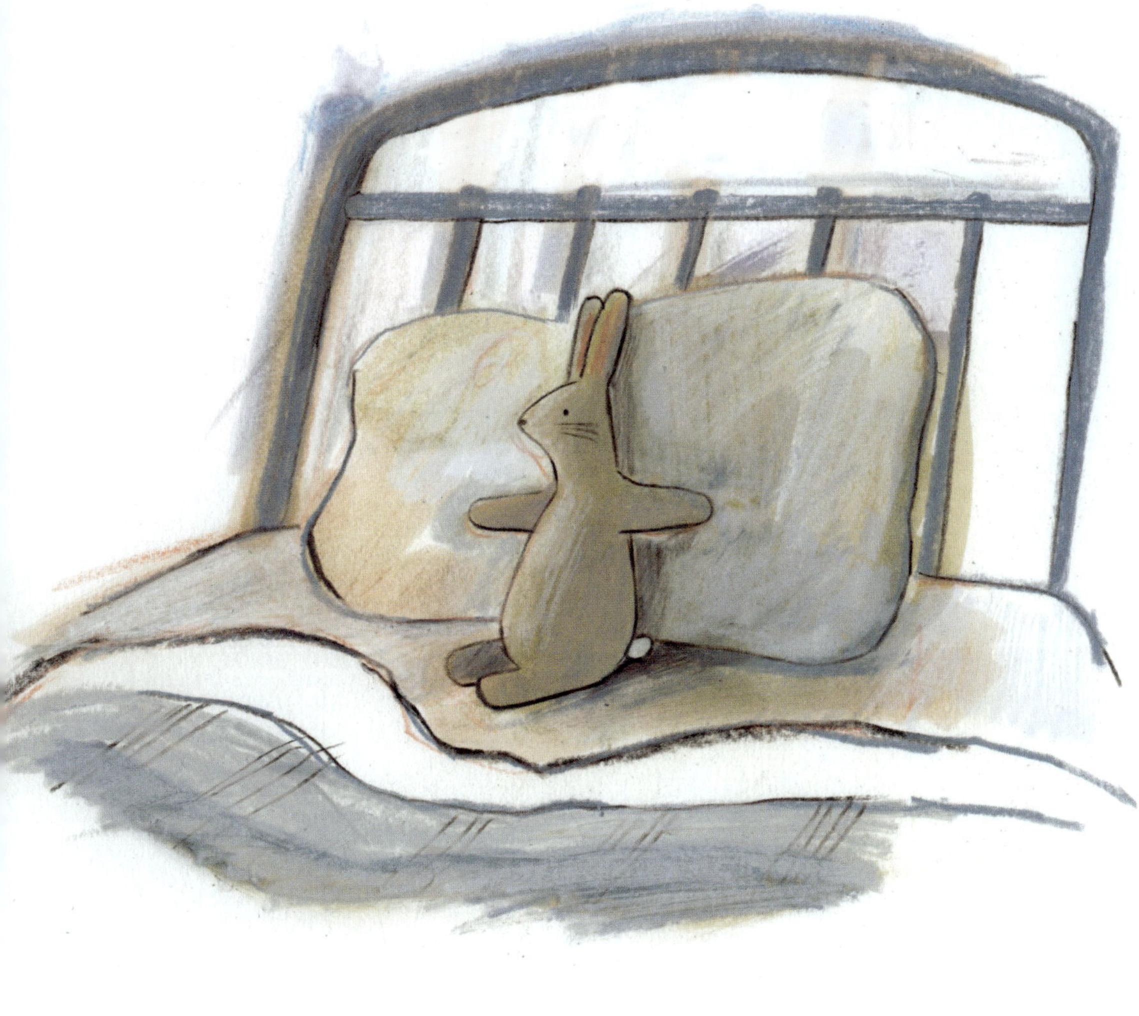

*Do not underestimate the power of being there:*
*your presence has huge value.*

*That night he was almost too happy to sleep, and so much love stirred in his little sawdust heart that it almost burst.*

Happiness often comes suddenly, in surprising moments and when least expected. Be open to these moments and mindful of their occurrence. Recognizing, acknowledging, and sharing them is important too.

Happiness is also about enjoying what you already have and it can take practice and moments of gratitude to truly recognize this.

So often, we anticipate the negative, which can inadvertently close us off to happiness. This mindset can be challenged by deliberately seeking out and noticing the positive in life—sometimes as simple as exchanging a smile with a fellow passenger as you board the bus.

*Actively choose happiness on a daily basis: it is not something "out there"—it is found within you.*

Near the house where they lived there was a wood … the Boy liked to go there after tea to play. He took the Velveteen Rabbit with him. One evening, while the Rabbit was lying there alone … he saw two strange beings creep out of the tall bracken near him.

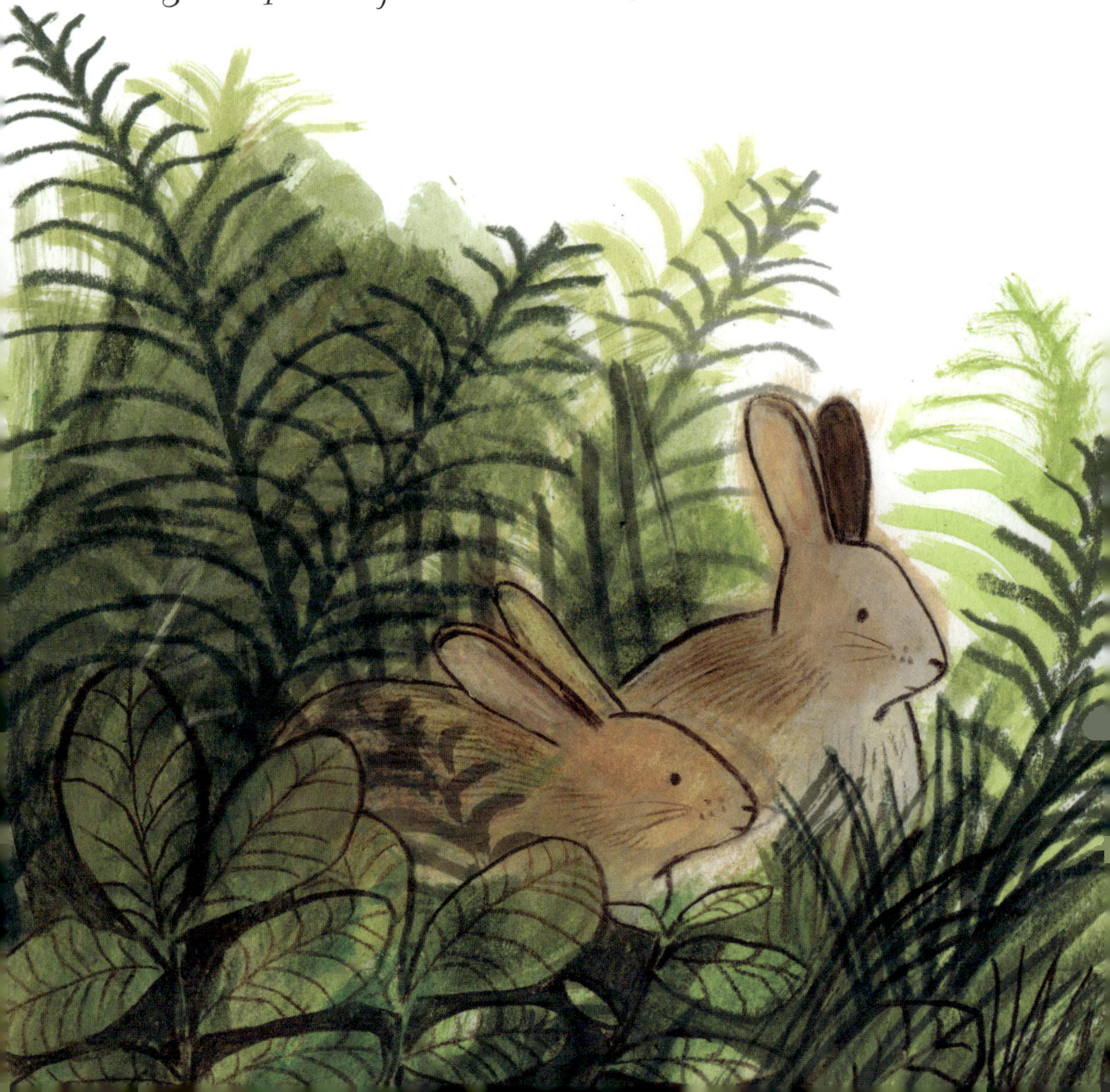

Some of life's lessons are simply about the daily practice of getting along with people who are different to us in some way. We may speak a different language, dress or look differently, or have a visible or hidden disability, but at heart our hopes and dreams are often very much the same.

How we approach new people or situations can be colored by expectations learnt in early life, and those can sometimes unconsciously prejudice our attitude.

It's good to be aware of this and keep an open mind; otherwise we may deny ourselves the opportunity to extend life's positive experiences. While it's OK to be cautious, don't close yourself off to life's possibilities.

*The choices you make tell people who you are.*

*'They were rabbits like himself, but quite furry and brand-new. They must have been very well made, for their seams didn't show at all ... They were evidently a new kind of rabbit altogether.*

Similar but different? Different but alike?

This is true of so many of us; we generally have more in common than not with other people. We all want to be valued and allowed to be ourselves, whatever form that might take.

When we only take others at face value, it's very easy to make assumptions about them, without knowing what their reality might be. Often, people cover up their insecurities, mask their worries, project their anxieties onto others, or conceal difficulties they don't want to share.

Bear this in mind when meeting those who seem different, and make responding with an open mind your default.

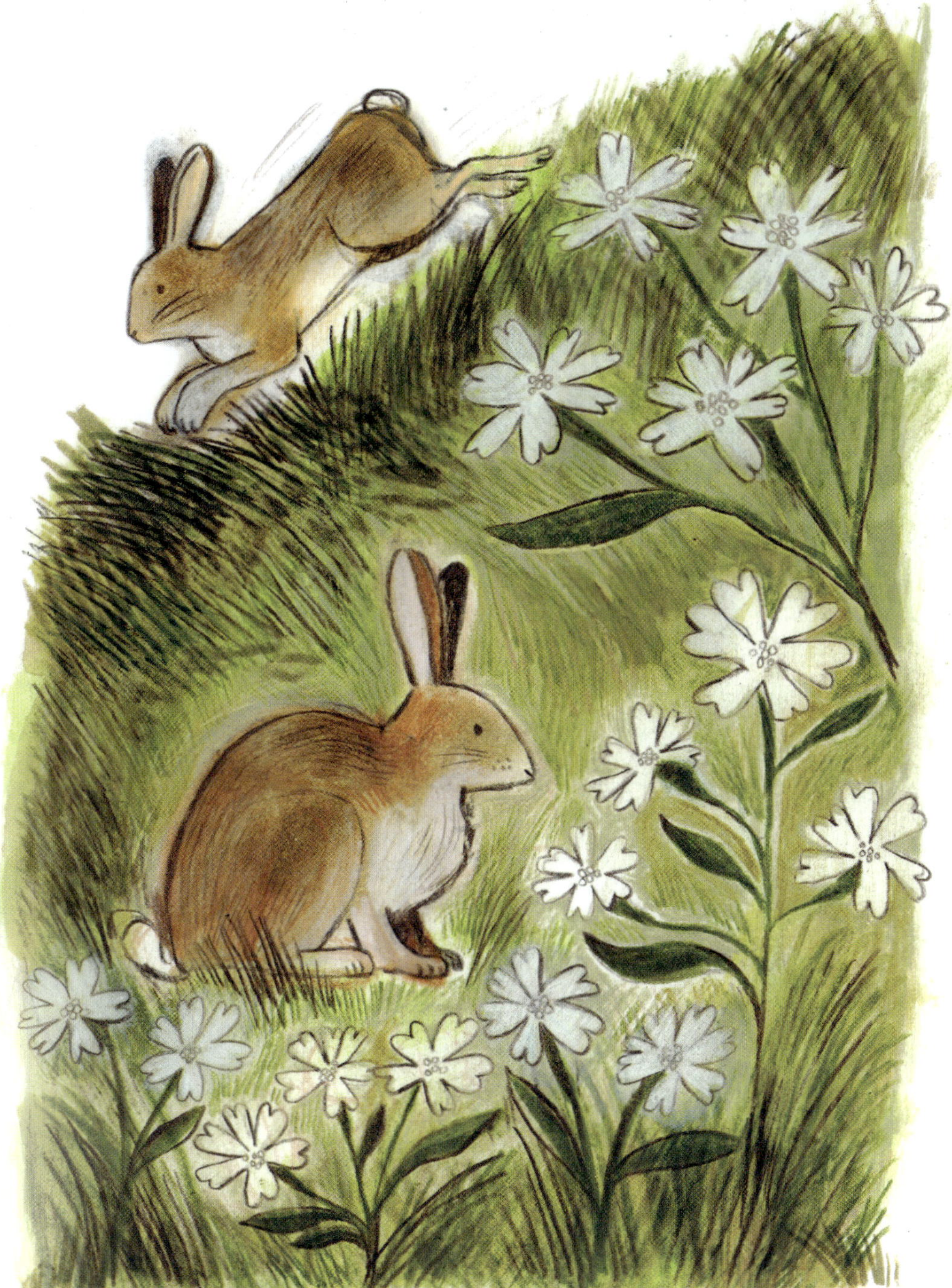

*In a world where you can be anything, be kind.*

*"Why don't you get up and play with us?" one of them asked. "I don't feel like it," said the Rabbit.*

Some days we can feel as if the world is an easy and accepting place; some days life can feel like a huge struggle and we may not want to attempt anything beyond the basics of our daily routine.

If we are feeling insecure or vulnerable or have taken a knock in some way, we might close ourselves off to new experiences, friends, or possibilities for fear of new hurt.

Pausing, taking stock, and evaluating what you do and don't want to attempt is fine, but it's good to think through what might be holding you back. Maybe talking it through with a trusted friend or taking a risk on something might help shift your perspective.

*Every single accomplishment comes from a decision to try.*

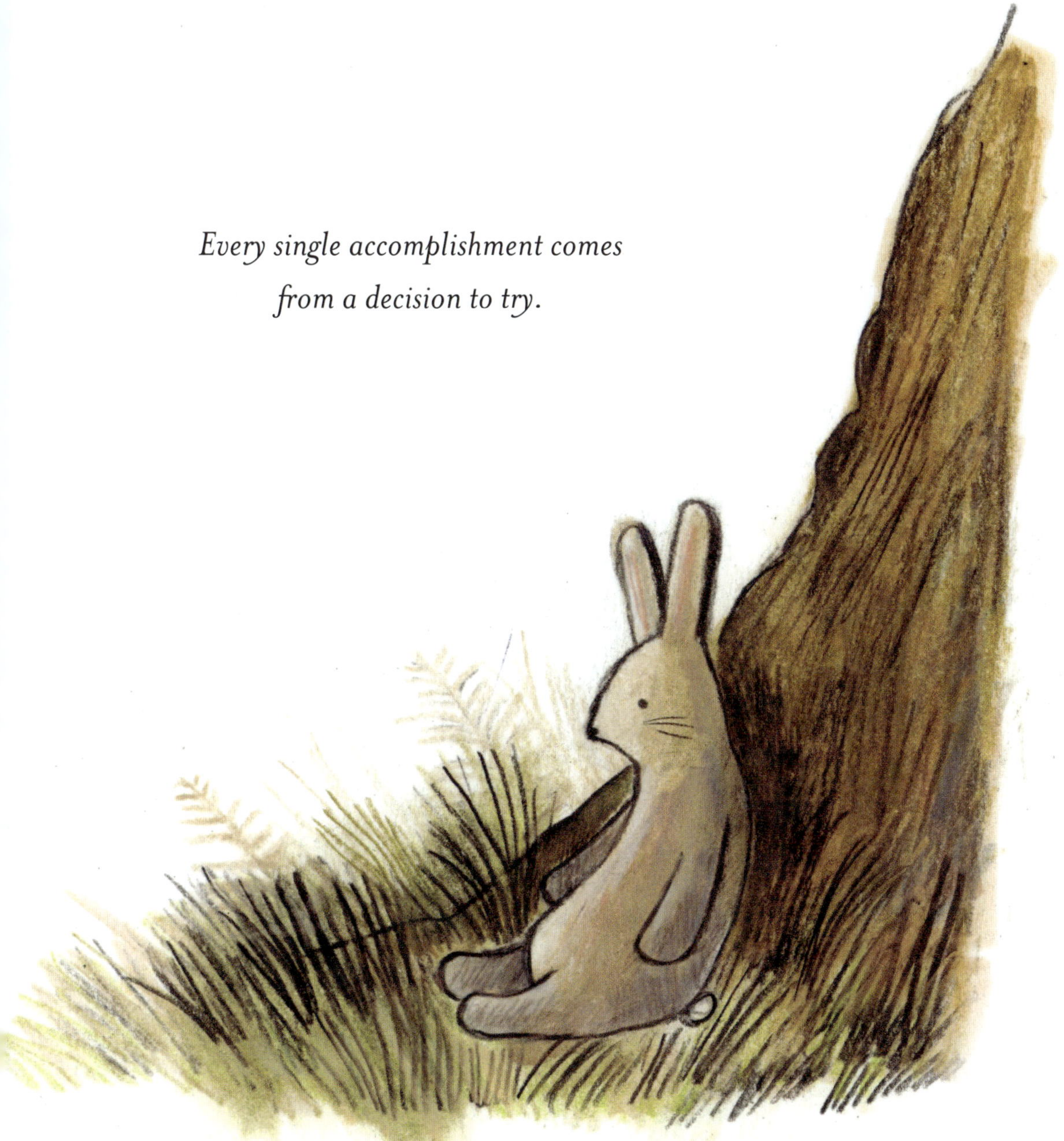

"Can you hop on your hind legs?" asked the furry rabbit ...

"I don't want to!" he said again ...

"He hasn't got any hind legs!" he called out. "Fancy a rabbit without any hind legs!" And he began to laugh.

"I have!" cried the little Rabbit. "I have got hind legs! I am sitting on them!"

When challenged it can be easy to retaliate with anxiety, especially in new situations. With people we don't know very well and on whom we'd like to make a good impression, we may find ourselves reacting in a way that is out of character.

Remember, whatever you are feeling, it will pass. Feeling something doesn't always make it true—but it can be a route to "a" truth. Feeling uncomfortable about something may help to work out and address the underlying causes of that feeling.

Like the little Rabbit who covered up his lack of hind legs with an excuse, we may cover up our feelings with a reaction. When this happens, take a moment to consider whether what you are feeling is true—your anxiety may be rooted in something in your past, rather than in your present.

*Bravery is not an absence of fear but finding the courage to push on through it.*

*"I don't like dancing," he said. "I'd rather sit still!" But all the while he was longing to dance, for a funny new tickly feeling ran through him, and he felt he would give anything in the world to be able to jump about like these rabbits did.*

Most of us have times when we fear making a fool of ourselves and are too embarrassed to give something a try, lacking the confidence to step out of our comfort zone. Choosing to sit something out while taking stock is fine, but you may lose more than you gain if you always choose to do this.

No one ever feels completely confident in new situations. When they arise, you may find it useful to remember past experiences in which you overcame nervousness to give something a try. If you have faced similar challenges before and the outcome was positive, remembering these occasions will remind you that you can manage this new one, transforming it into a challenge to be enjoyed.

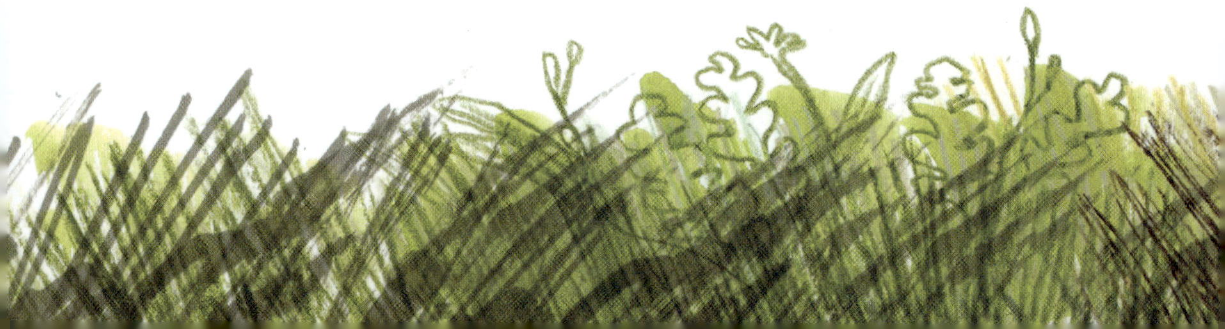

*In order to find yourself, you may have to risk losing yourself for a time.*

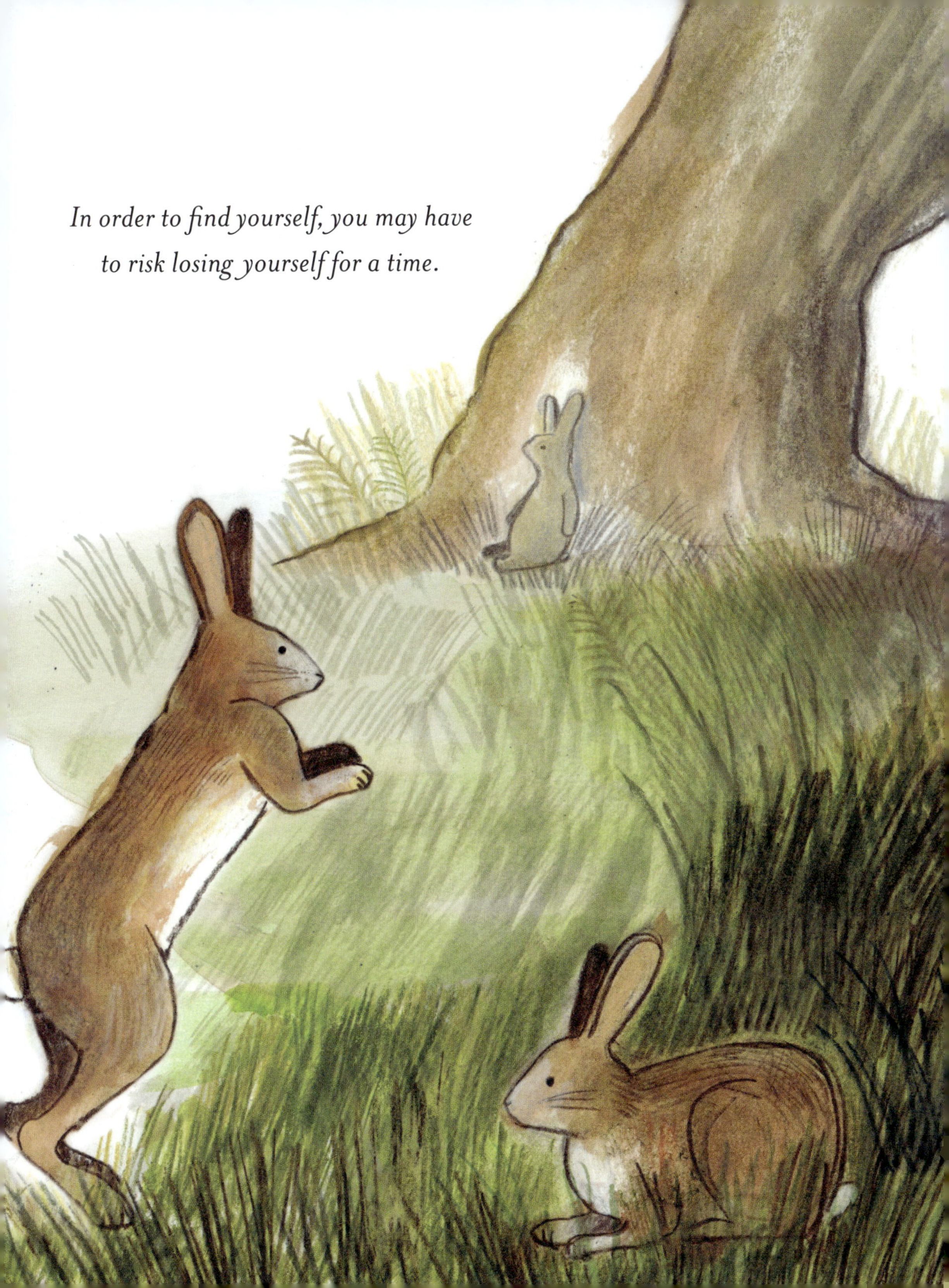

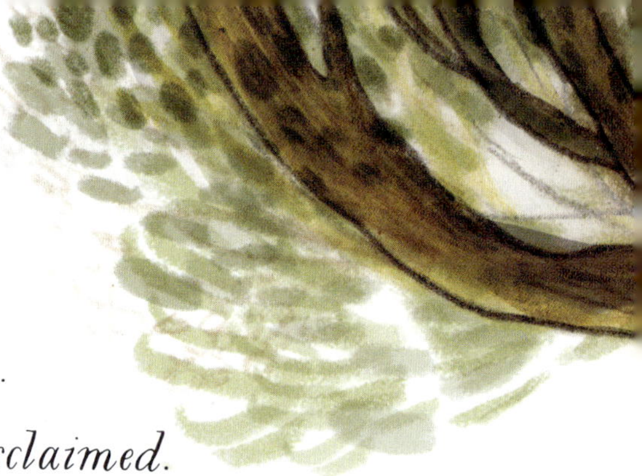

*The strange rabbit stopped dancing, and came quite close ...*
*"He doesn't smell right!" He exclaimed.*
*"He isn't a rabbit at all! He isn't Real!"*
*"I am Real!" said the little Rabbit.*
*"I am Real! The Boy said so!"*

Some days our self-confidence is so challenged by something that happens to us, it can leave us feeling unsure or undermined. A passing comment, an unexpected reaction, or a response you didn't anticipate can make you feel insecure.

This may make you question your own thoughts and beliefs or make you feel like an imposter. At these times, it's important to identify whether this is really the case or just your inner critic sabotaging your confidence.

This is when building resilience can help. Don't ruminate over what's happened but identify the key issue that has upset you, address it, then move on.

Here, the little Rabbit is reminded that someone who loves him has told him he is real, and that internalized belief now stands him in good stead.

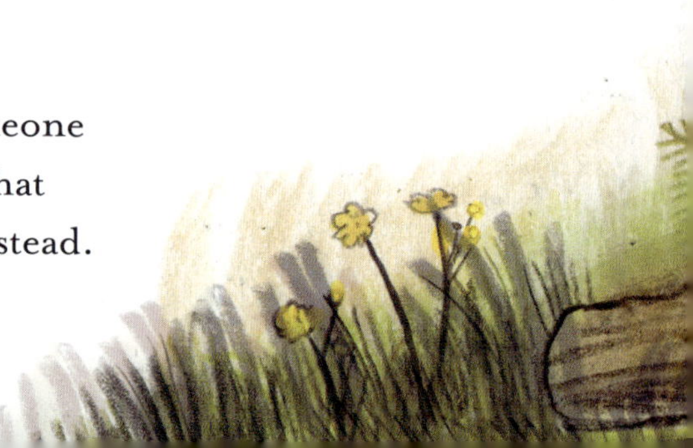

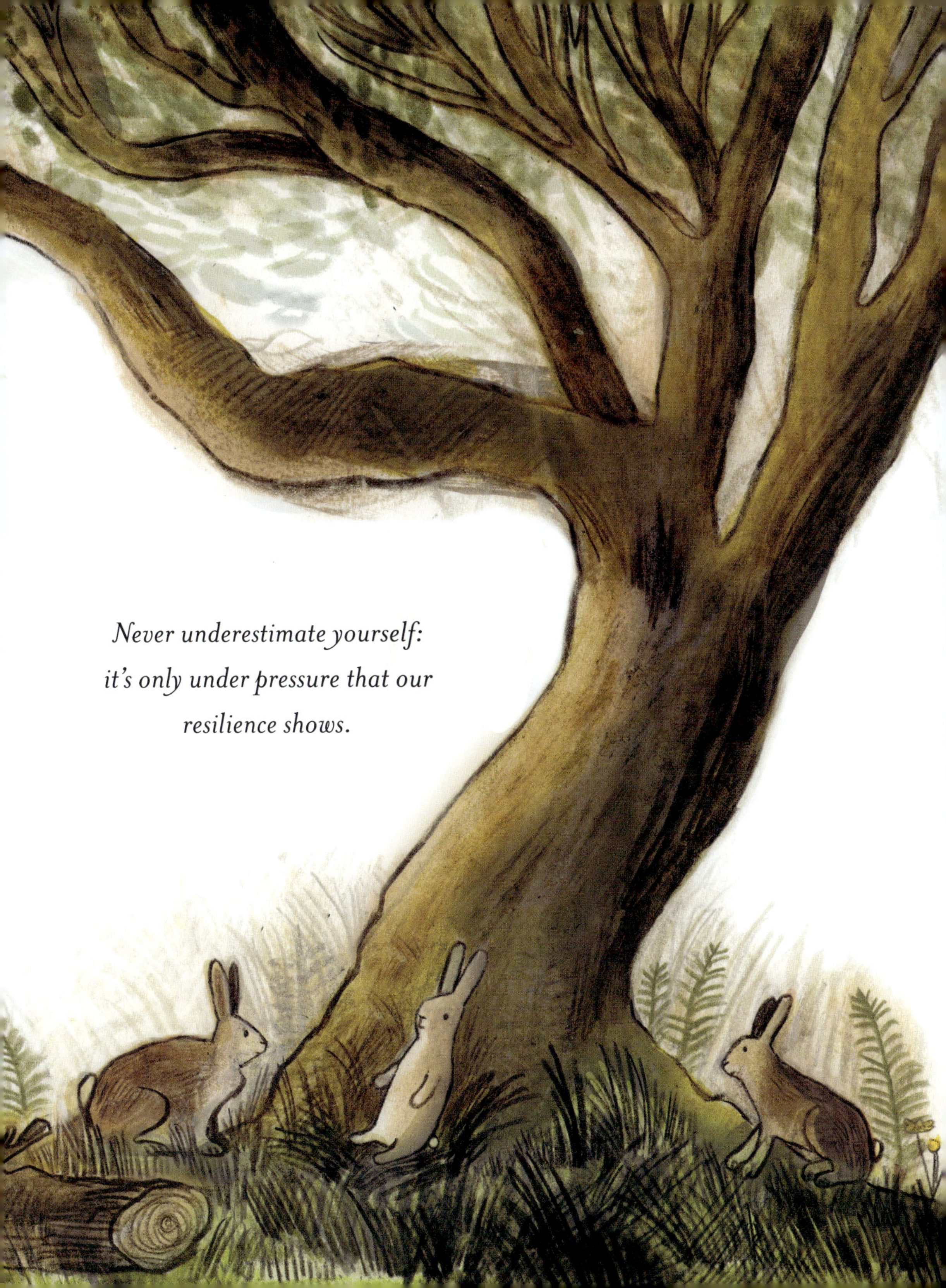

*Never underestimate yourself:*
*it's only under pressure that our*
*resilience shows.*

*"Oh dear!" he thought. "Why did they run away like that? Why couldn't they stop and talk to me?"*

It's only ever possible to manage our own feelings, responses, and actions—not anyone else's.

You are not responsible for other people's choices or decisions, only for your own. When something happens that you didn't anticipate or expect, hang on to the reality of your experience, rather than assume you're at fault in some way.

This is important if you are ever at the blunt end of someone else's behavior or gaslighting. Check the truth of your experience, rather than trying to second guess theirs. People do all sorts of things for their own reasons, but we cannot be responsible for any behavior other than our own.

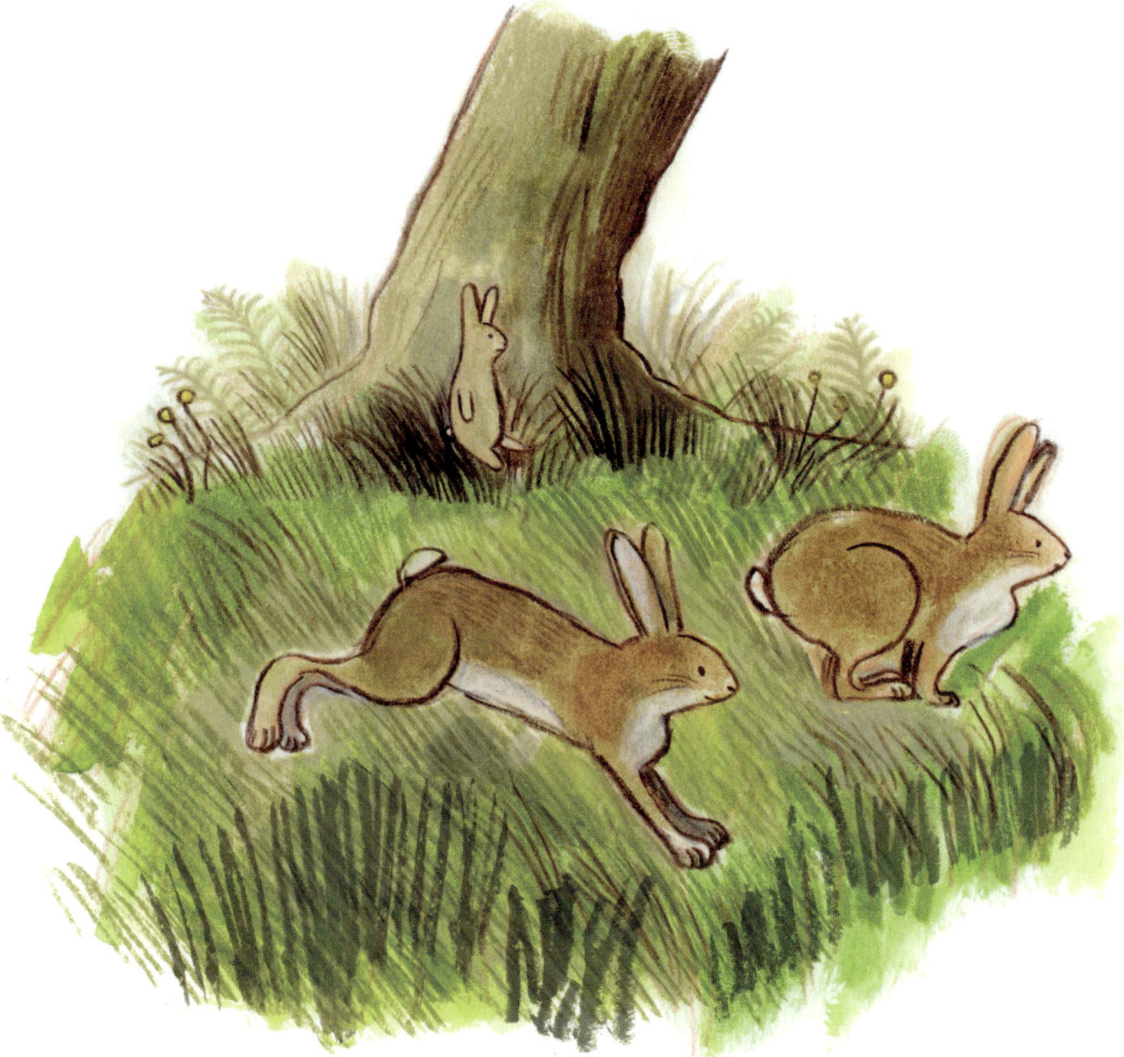

*Let your truth be your guide.*

*Weeks passed, and the little Rabbit grew very old and shabby ... he scarcely looked like a rabbit any more, except to the Boy. To him he was always beautiful ... because the nursery magic had made him Real, and when you are Real, shabbiness doesn't matter.*

We sometimes attach enormous value to external appearances, but it's the exploration of our internal life that helps us develop who we are.

Socrates said, "The unexamined life is not worth living," meaning that it is important to pay attention to your thoughts and feelings, how they impact on the choices you make, and on the actions you take.

It's not always easy to see the beauty in our lives, especially if we make comparisons with those we feel are more attractive or successful than us. Remember that the only thoughts worth investing any value in are your own, so make sure they're positive.

*If the grass looks greener on the other side,*

*water the grass on your side.*

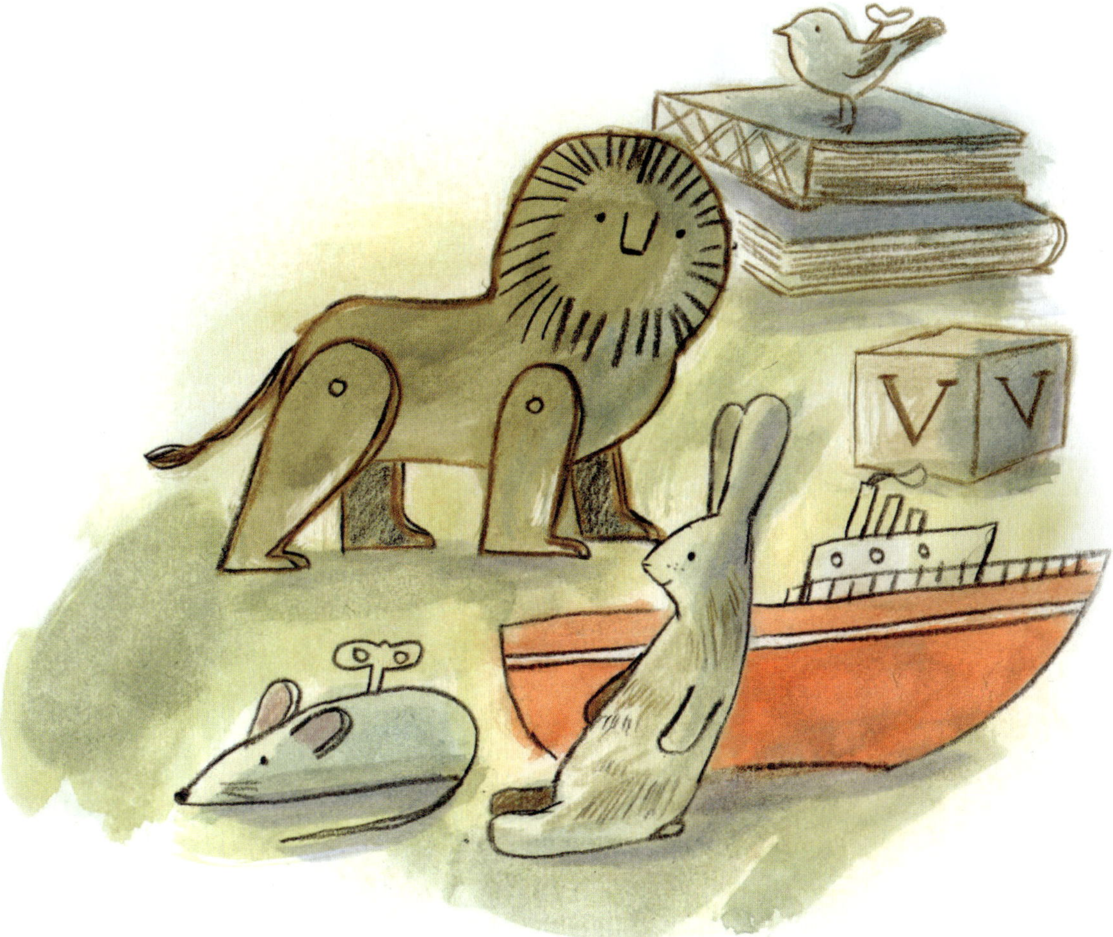

*And then, one day, the Boy was ill.*

Adversity comes in all sorts of shapes and sizes and no one goes through life without experiencing it. While managing adversity can challenge you in new ways, you probably already have life skills to help you—instead, look to those around you to support you.

Acknowledging and accepting what has happened is a first step, whether adversity has happened to you or to someone you love. Focus on the immediate hours ahead rather than too far into the future, and manage your response with compassion while you wait to adjust.

Ground yourself in the knowledge that change happens and all things must pass.

*Adversity can be a wake-up call to make the changes you want in life.*

*It was a long weary time, for the Boy was too ill to play, and the little Rabbit found it rather dull with nothing to do all day long. But he snuggled down patiently, and looked forward to the time when the Boy should be well again ... And presently the fever turned and the Boy got better.*

Not everything in life can be fast paced and exciting; sometimes we need to take things slowly. If our energy flags for any reason, it can be a good opportunity to reflect and review how things are working out for us. Recovery can also allow time to revise and refocus our hopes and dreams.

Nothing ever stays the same. Change always affords us an opportunity to reconsider how things are and how we might like them to be. Then we can take steps towards realizing those positive changes.

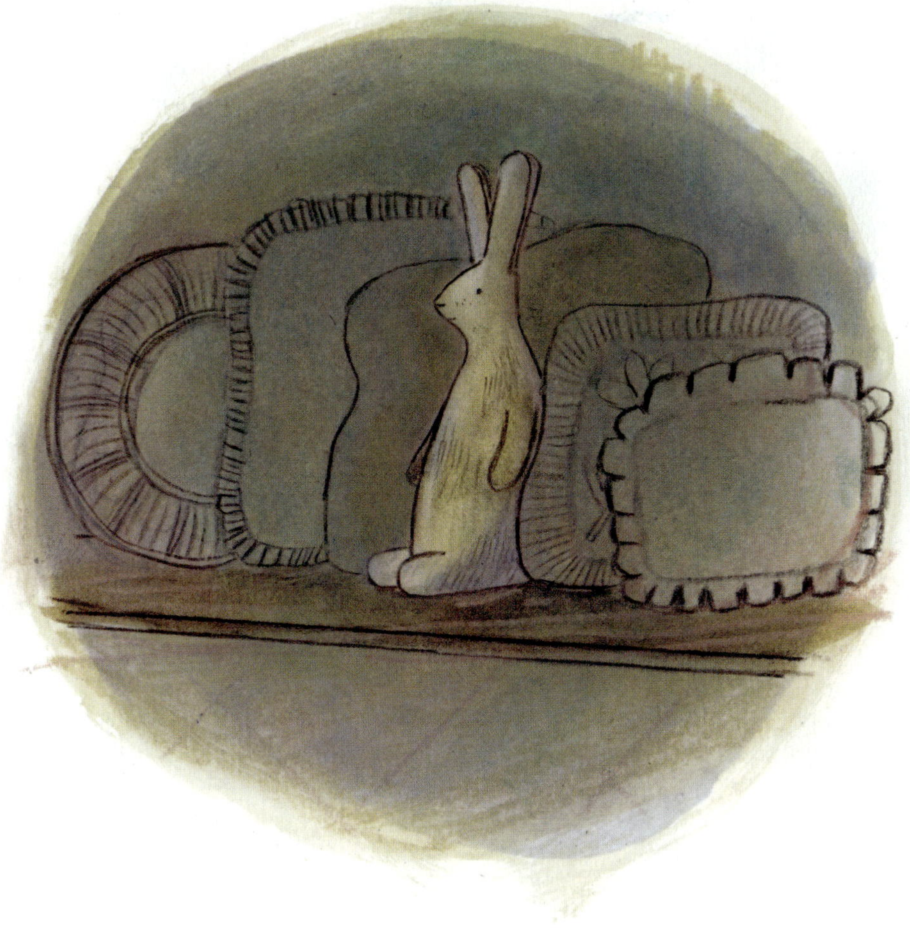

*For your plans to succeed, you'll need
to constantly adapt, revise, and change.*

*"How about this old Bunny?" Nana asked. "That?" said the doctor. "Why, it's a mass of scarlet fever germs! Burn it at once."*

Sometimes we need to do something radical to make changes and it may not be immediately obvious what.

We don't need to burn all our bridges, but we can look at the different directions we might consider and work out which of these most closely aligns with our long-term goals.

Sometimes it's just a question of trying differently, not harder, to affect the change you need to make. Take your time to consider your options, shift your perspective, and wait until it's clear to you what the next step might be.

*Those things that excite you are a clue to your life's purpose.*

*And so the little Rabbit was put into a sack with the old picture-books and a lot of rubbish, and carried out to the end of the garden.*

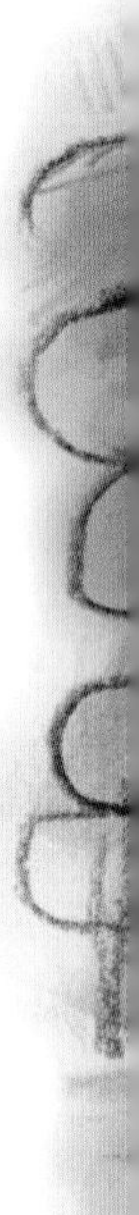

Often, endings are actually new beginnings, even if they don't feel like it at the time. But remember, the excitement of New Year's Eve marks the ending of the old year as much as the beginning of the new one.

While beginnings feel exciting, they can also feel uncertain and frightening. In fact, excitement can also feel like fear, and vice versa. Even if the same racing heart and breathlessness is for something positive, these physical feelings can sometimes trigger anxiety. It can be useful to identify this for what it is—anticipatory nerves—then, calm and ground your body and mind in preparation for the next step.

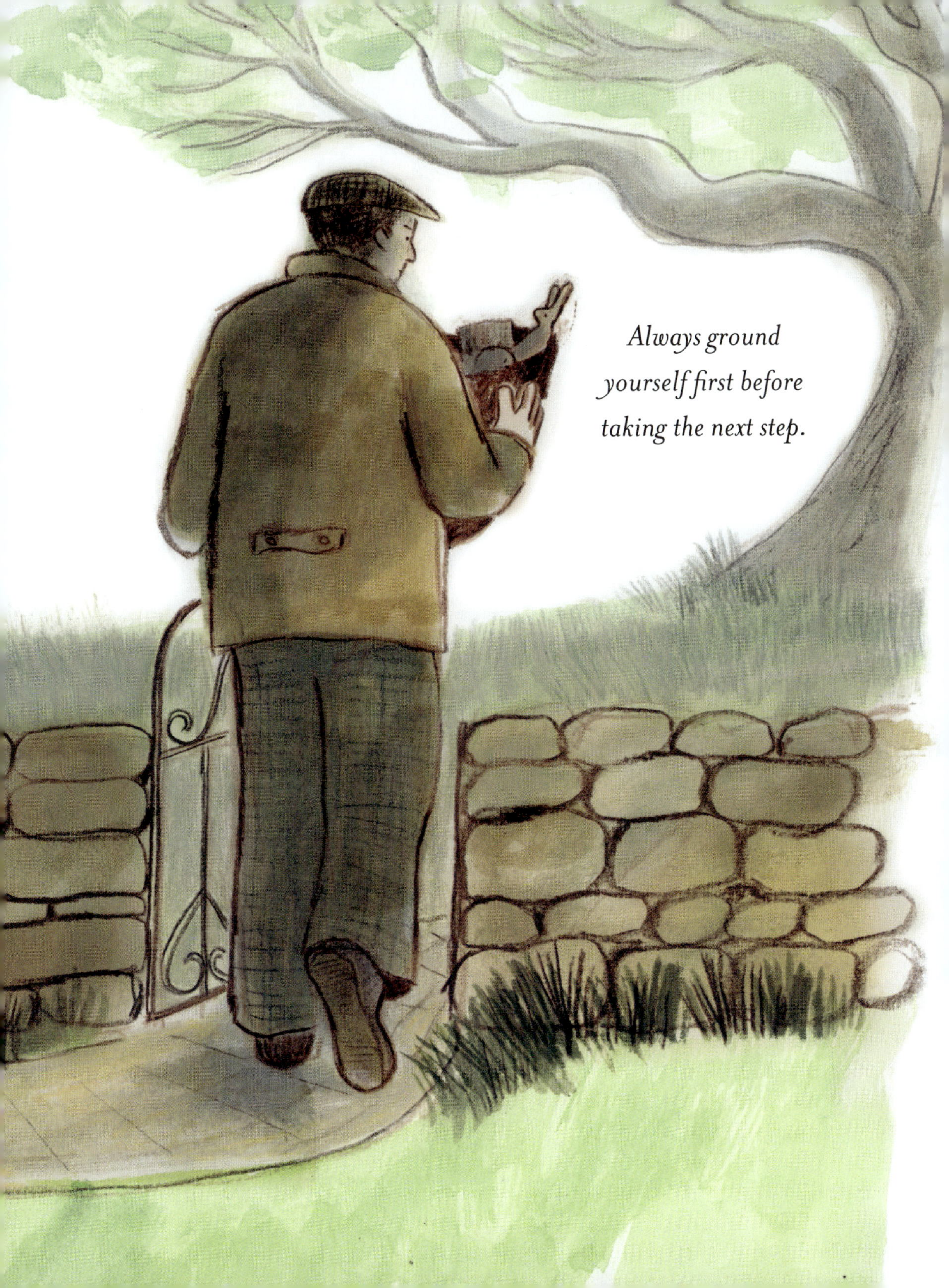

*Always ground yourself first before taking the next step.*

*And while the Boy was asleep, dreaming of the seaside, the little Rabbit lay among the old picture-books ... and he felt very lonely.*

Even in the middle of a crowd we can feel lonely, particularly if we are wrestling with change or uncertainty. Loneliness can isolate us—but this is exactly the time to seek meaningful connections with others, either close friends in whom you can confide or through activities that refresh our emotional attachments.

Many people find this tricky, especially when circumstances change—moving locations, starting a new school or job, or having a baby, for example, are all times we need to draw on inner resources. Remembering previous occasions when difficulties were overcome reassures us that we can and will cope, making loneliness a temporary experience that we can manage and overcome.

*Don't immediately run from occasional solitude; it will often yield its own reward.*

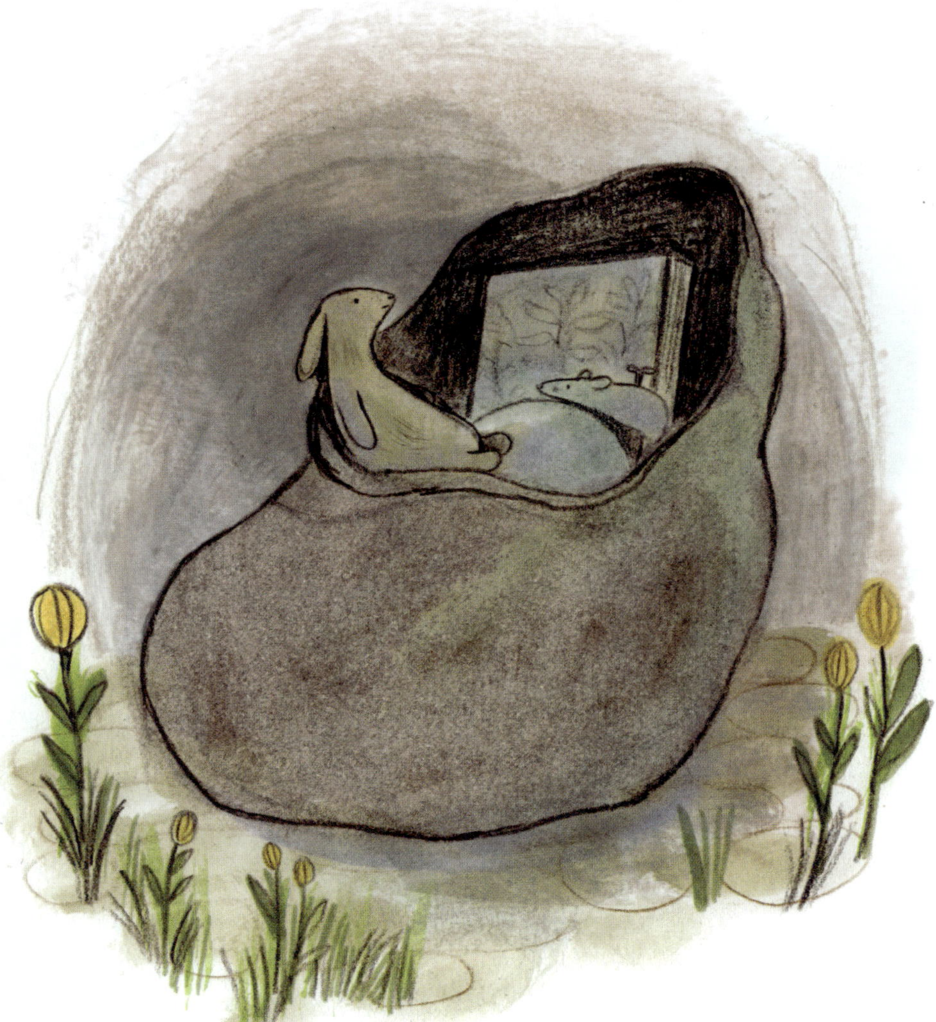

*He thought of the Skin Horse, so wise and gentle, and all that he had told him. Of what use was it to be loved and lose one's beauty and become Real if it all ended like this?*

Loving and accepting ourselves is how we become real. That means accepting the things we don't like about ourselves—perhaps working to change them, but also loving ourselves unconditionally. If we put conditions on how we might be worthy of love, we reduce its possibilities.

Discovering these internal truths will reveal the authenticity of our unique existence. In loving our true and real selves, it becomes possible to extend that same love and acceptance towards others and into the world. And finding this reality is a good place to reach for.

*When in doubt, pause and take stock. The right answer will often reveal itself given time.*

*And a tear, a real tear, trickled down his little shabby velvet nose and fell to the ground.*

Real feelings elicit real tears; feeling sad shows us we are human.

There will be times when we feel at our lowest ebb, as if we are stuck and alone, have no agency, and there is nothing we can do. When this happens, think about other times when you felt frustrated and unsure, and remember what you did about it.

We often fear change, but if we reflect on past experiences and what we learned from them to get through a difficult patch it can really help. What did you do? Who did you confide in? Did you wait it out or did you seek help?

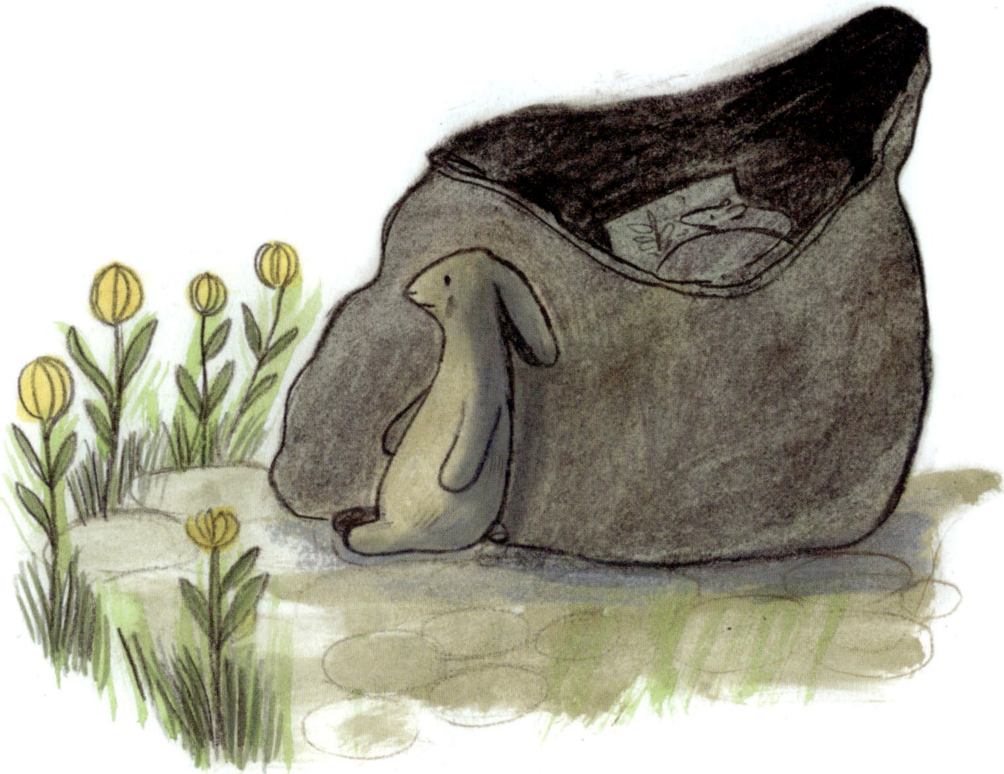

*It's at its lowest ebb that the tide always turns.*

*"I am the nursery magic Fairy," she said. "I take care of all the playthings that the children have loved. When they are old and worn out and the children don't need them any more, then I come and take them away with me and turn them into Real."*

In your heart you may know that you need to make changes, but it may not be immediately obvious how to do this to your best advantage. How can you be your own magic fairy and identify your next step?

It may be a moment of inspiration that brings you clarity or it may be a hard-won process of trial and error, but that moment of transformation doesn't come from nowhere. It comes from those lessons learned through your own efforts, relationships, and authenticity. Trust this process—you can be confident it's based on investments you've already made.

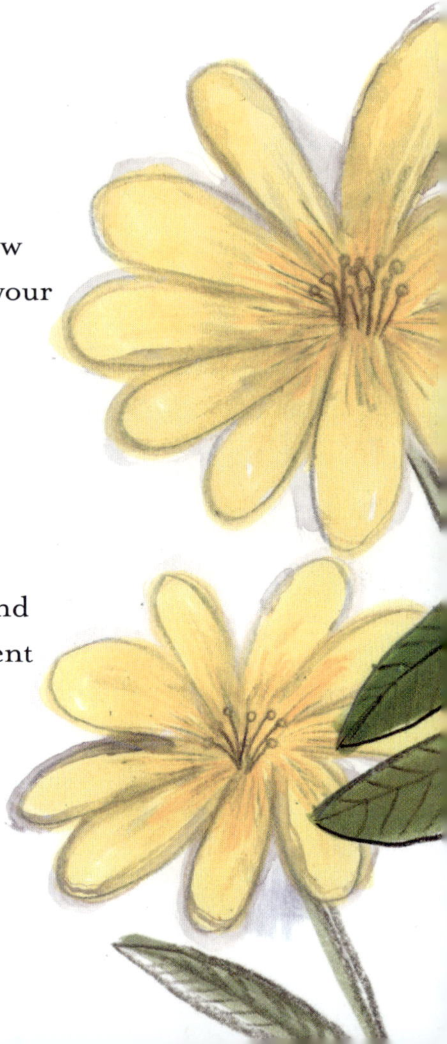

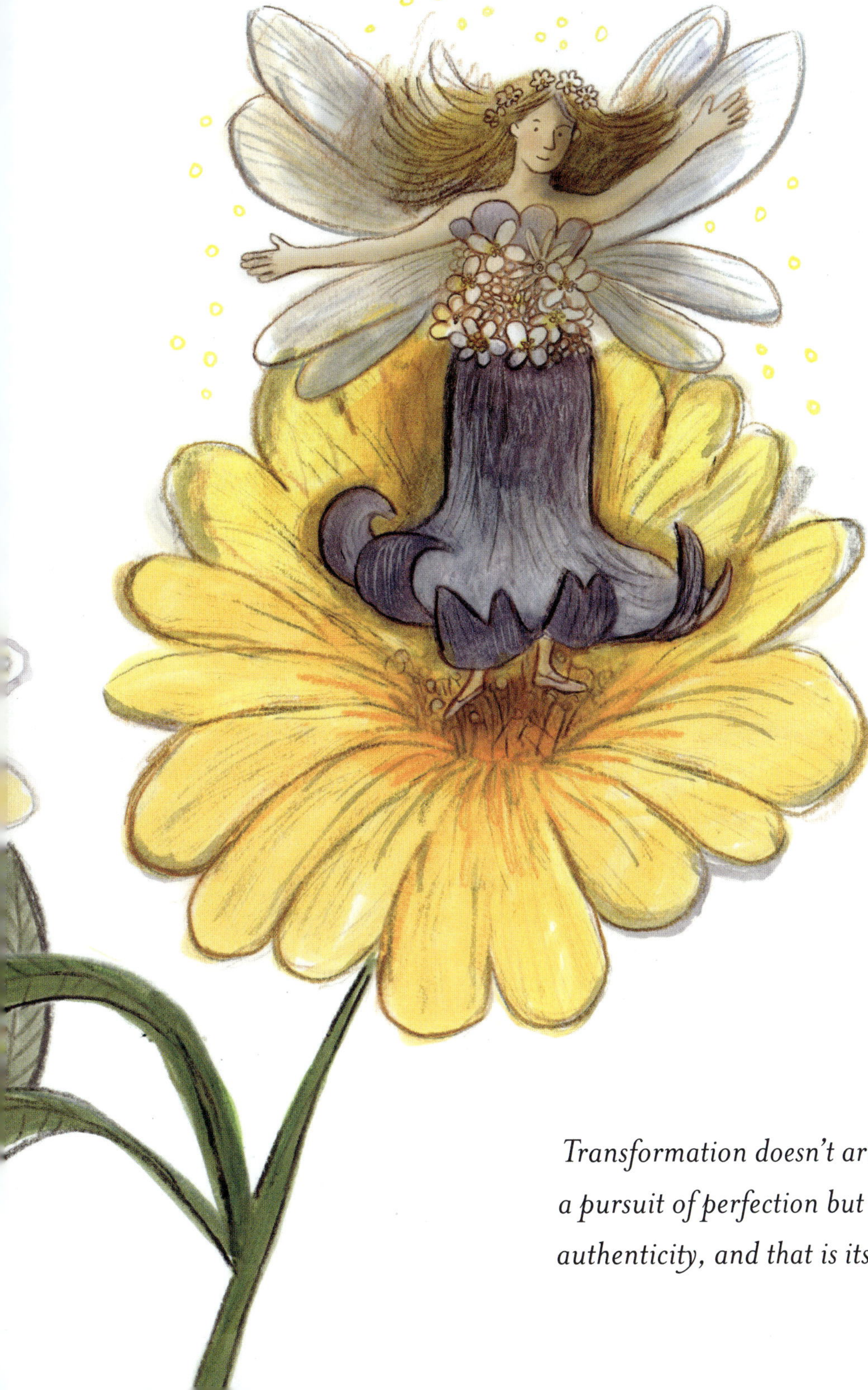

*Transformation doesn't arise from a pursuit of perfection but through authenticity, and that is its beauty.*

*"Wasn't I Real before?" asked the little Rabbit.*

*"You were Real to the Boy," the Fairy said, "because he loved you. Now you shall be Real to everyone." And she held the little Rabbit close in her arms and flew with him into the wood.*

Sometimes we don't realize how far we've traveled until we arrive. Other times, it is those around us who reflect back the reality of the journey we've been on—through them we can recognize what we've achieved in pursuit of our dreams and aims.

The support of others in realizing a dream can be wonderful, and we in turn can support those we care about. Often a journey can be rather lonely without the reality of a loving community, so it's good to invest time and energy in connections—those friendships and relationships that can help us thrive.

*When you show up as your most authentic self, it's easier to foster connections and relationships that enable real change.*

*In the open glade between the tree trunks the wild rabbits danced ... "I've brought you a new playfellow," the Fairy said. "You must be very kind to him and teach him all he needs to know ... for he is going to live with you forever and ever!"*

Forever and ever can feel like a long time—as if you've got all the time in the world. And while the stepping stones of your journey may not be immediately obvious as you move forward, rest assured they will reveal themselves as surely as day follows night, as long as you take the next step, and the next.

Each stepping stone is a building block on which you create your future, each experience a learning opportunity that will help realize your dreams. As your confidence in yourself builds, so too will your future.

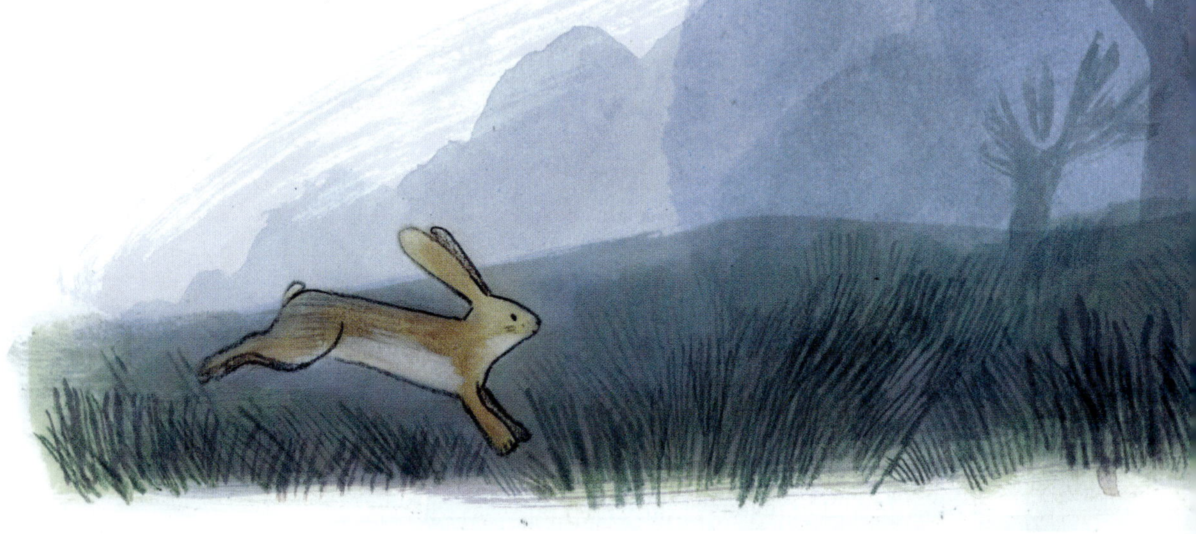

*The future always has a place for you,*
*so step into it with certainty.*

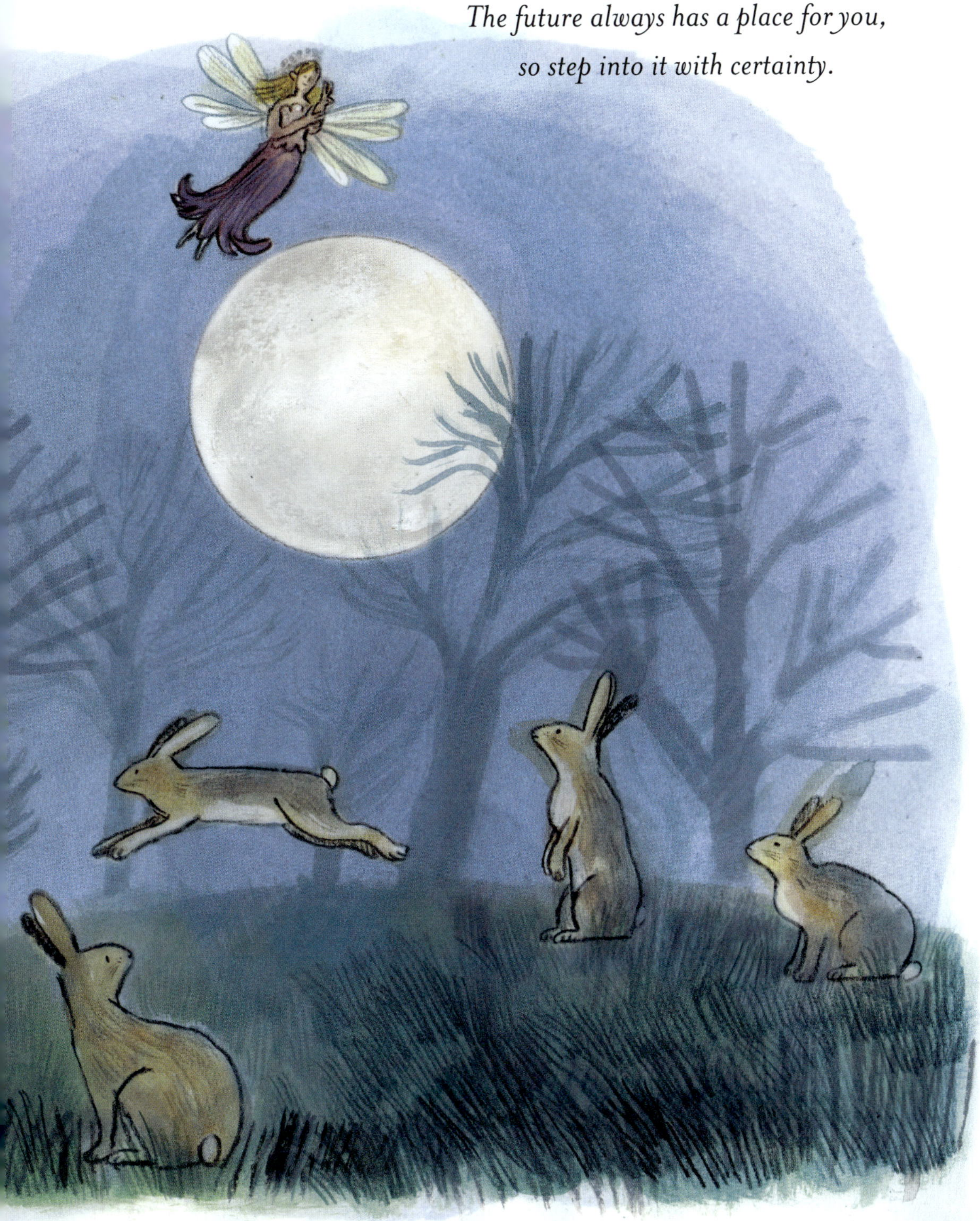

*And she kissed the little Rabbit again and put him down on the grass.*

Ground yourself. When life feels challenging or a struggle, take a moment to connect with what grounds you, especially at the beginning of something new.

You may not feel completely confident or sure of your next step but reminding yourself of the progress you've already made and how far you've come in pursuit of your dreams, will help ground you. Then you can take your next steps with greater confidence.

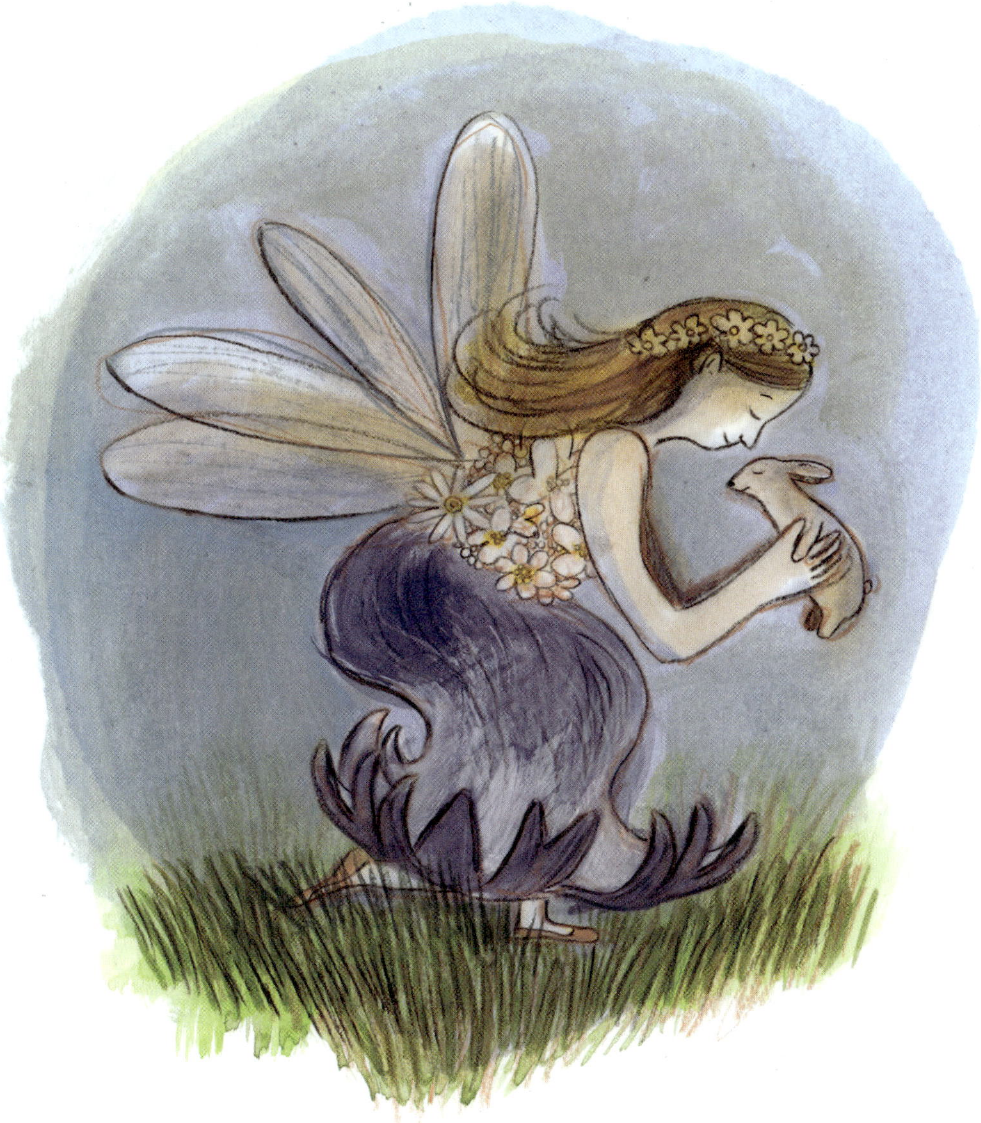

*Start with what you have; do with it what you can.*

*"Run and play, little Rabbit."*

Play isn't just for children, it's also been proven to be essential for the emotional health of adults too. Exercising imagination and playfulness can enhance our mood, help us solve problems, and release the brain from the ruminations of worry that can fuel anxiety.

Sharing playful times, creating memories, and laughing together, can sustain us long after the moment has passed. Wellbeing is enhanced by both emotional and physical activity, together they can lift the soul. Happiness is rooted in wellbeing. Invest in play times, whatever works for you, to create the life balance your happiness needs.

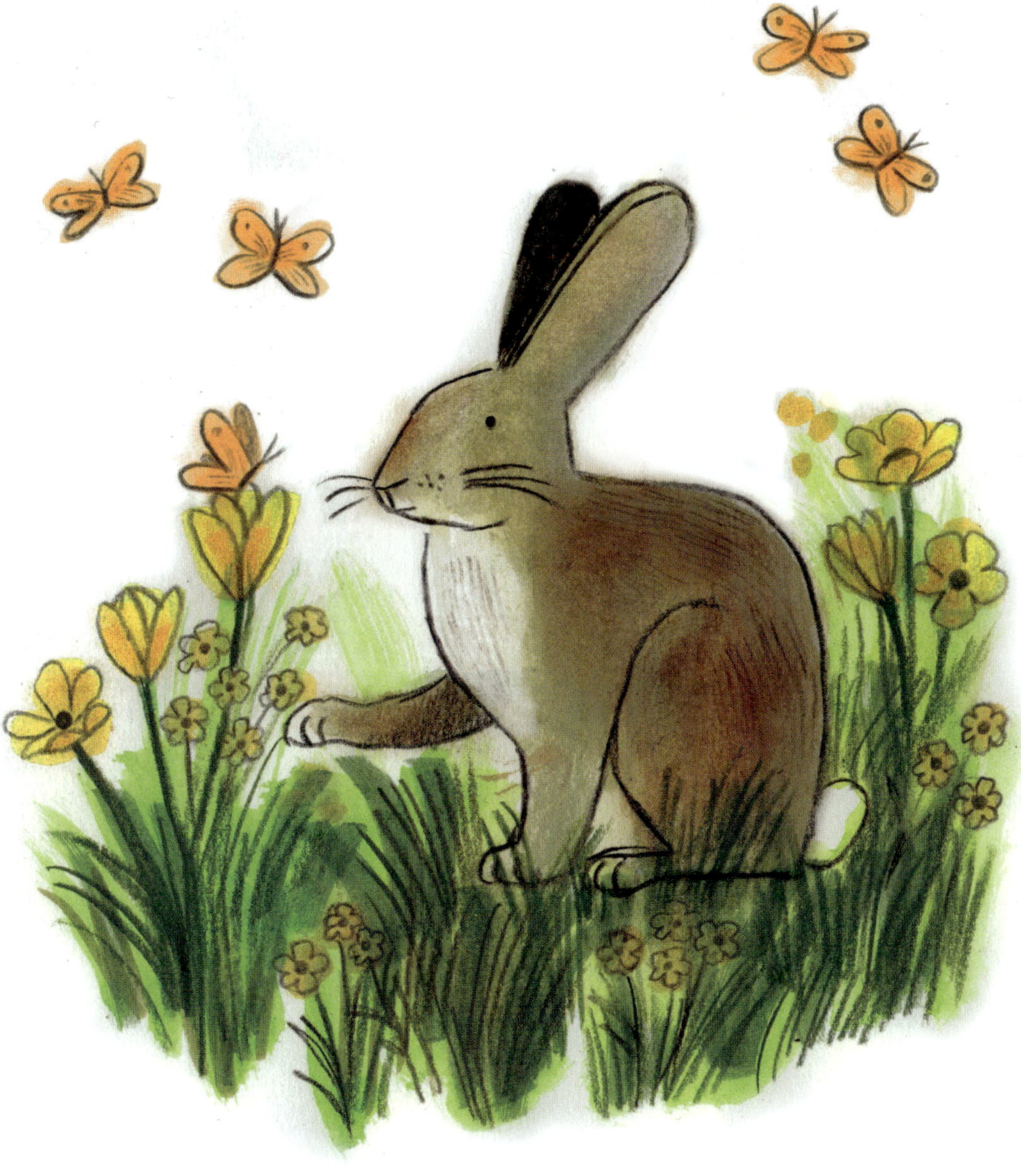

*You are not responsible for the happiness of others, only your own; but your happiness can help contribute to theirs.*

*He did not know that when the Fairy kissed him that last time she had changed him altogether.*

The process of becoming who we truly are is often more apparent to an outsider than ourselves.

Remember when you were a child, and someone who hadn't seen you for a while would say, "Haven't you grown?" Inner growth of our mind and spirit may be less obvious to others, but it shows in our actions and interactions, and this becomes more evident as we become adults.

We don't develop our confidence and sense of self in a vacuum, but in response to our relationships, surroundings, and circumstances, so whenever possible choose those that nourish you.

The little Rabbit was emotionally nourished by his relationship with the Boy and the Wise Horse, whose love was just as instrumental in helping him become real as was the Fairy's magic kiss.

*The wings of transformation come from patience and struggle: remember this every time you see a butterfly.*

*He was a Real Rabbit at last,*
*at home with the other rabbits.*

When we find our tribe, it can feel like coming home. This can take time and, for some of us, a lifetime. But it is always possible. What matters is staying open to opportunities and exploring what feels authentically right for you.

We may have spent time conforming to other people's ideas of what we should be or how we should live our lives, and it may take trial and error to find a home for our heart and soul. But this journey of exploration can be a gift in itself; each day of that journey is a blessing that allows us the time we need to become the best of ourselves.

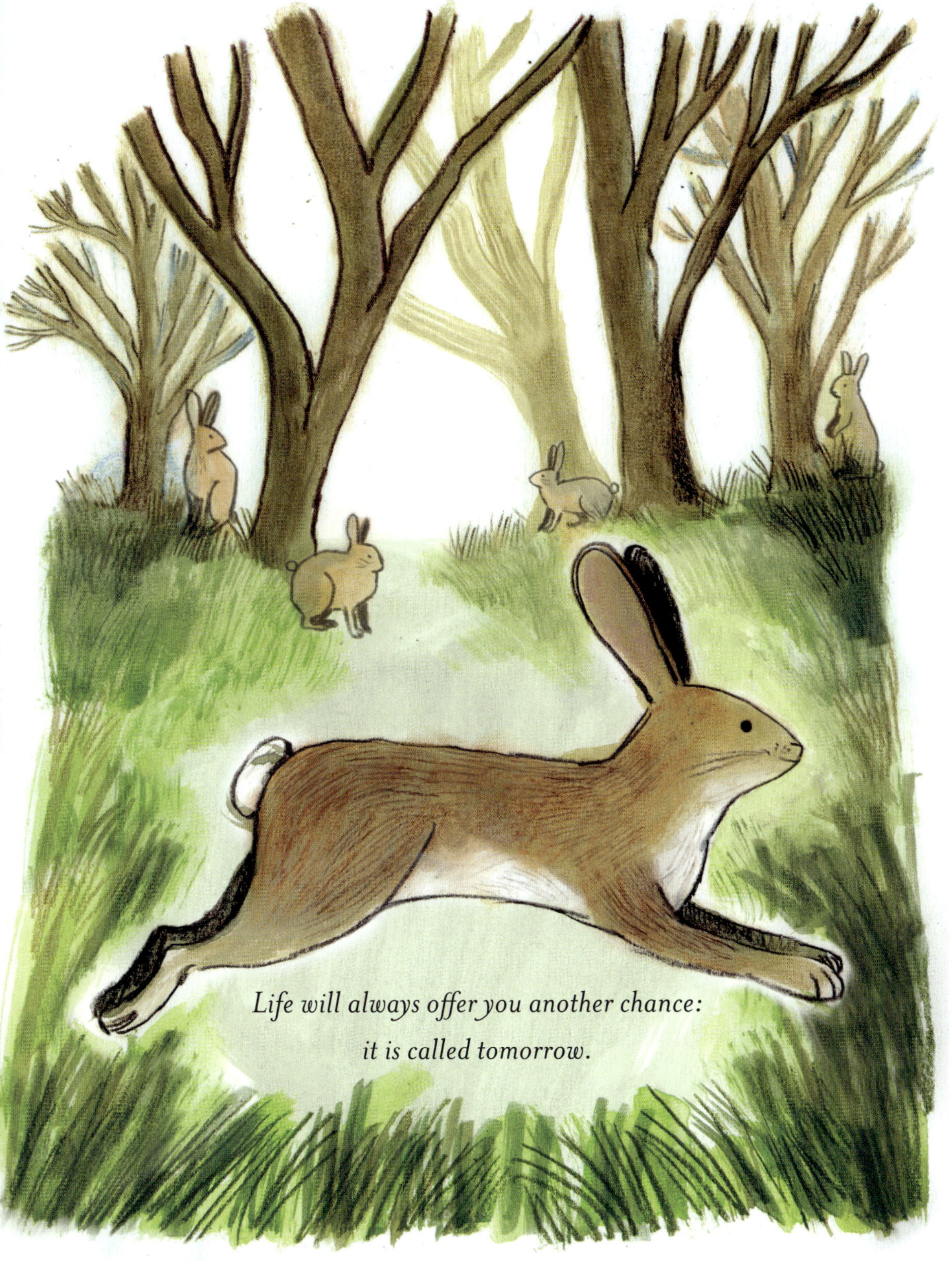

*Life will always offer you another chance:*
*it is called tomorrow.*

*In the Spring, when the days grew warm and sunny, the Boy went out to play in the wood behind the house. And while he was playing, two rabbits crept out from the bracken and peeped at him ... "Why, he looks just like my old Bunny that was lost!"*

Memories are an important part of who we are. Creating good memories, sharing them, and enjoying them can remind us of what really matters. This isn't about living in the past, but embracing positive lessons learned, using them to create resilience and authenticity, and recognizing what was required of us to become our "real" selves.

Internalizing those positive feelings gives us a reference point, a gentle reminder that we are authentic and resilient, and can exercise self-compassion toward ourselves and others.

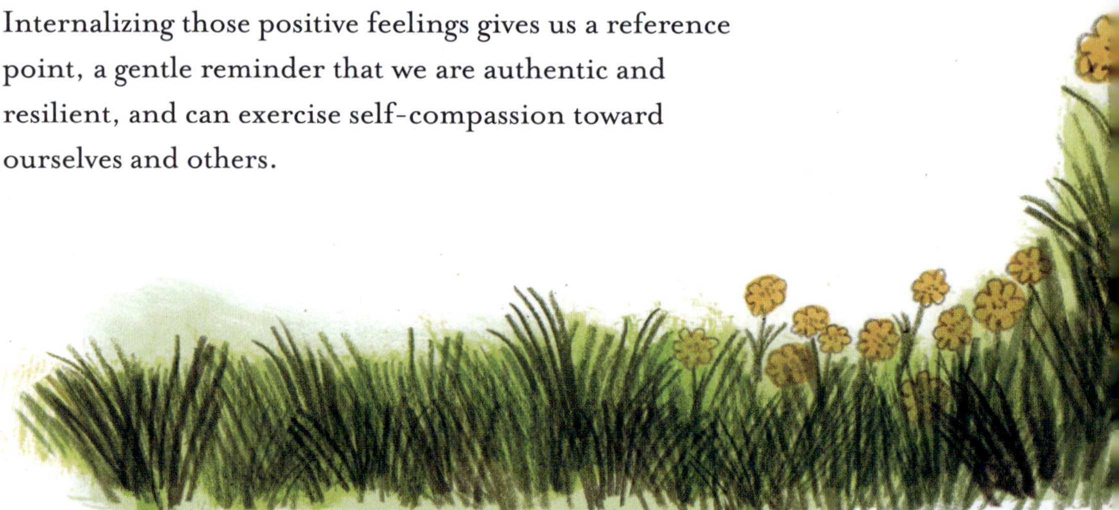

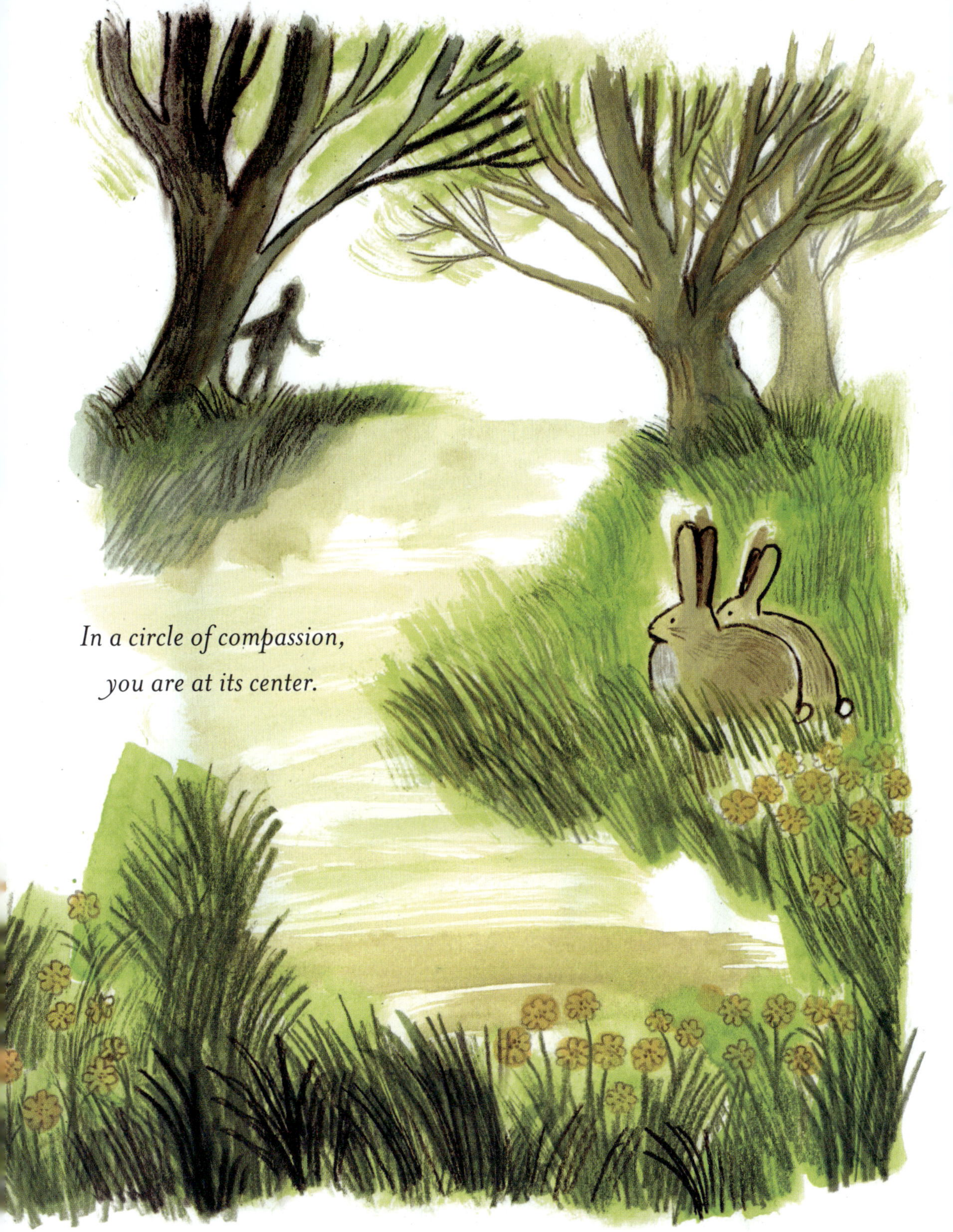

*In a circle of compassion,*
*you are at its center.*

*But he never knew that it really was his own Bunny, come back to look at the child who had first helped him to be Real.*

Connections made for the right reasons last forever.

Long after those physical connections have ceased, their memories can fortify us. You may have had a grandparent who had been your special advocate and safe haven, who gave you unconditional love, and even with their physical presence gone, the strength of their belief in you remains.

Whoever was your good parent, mentor, or friend, will have taught you that you matter, and this will stay in your heart forever. Their belief in you is real, just as you are.

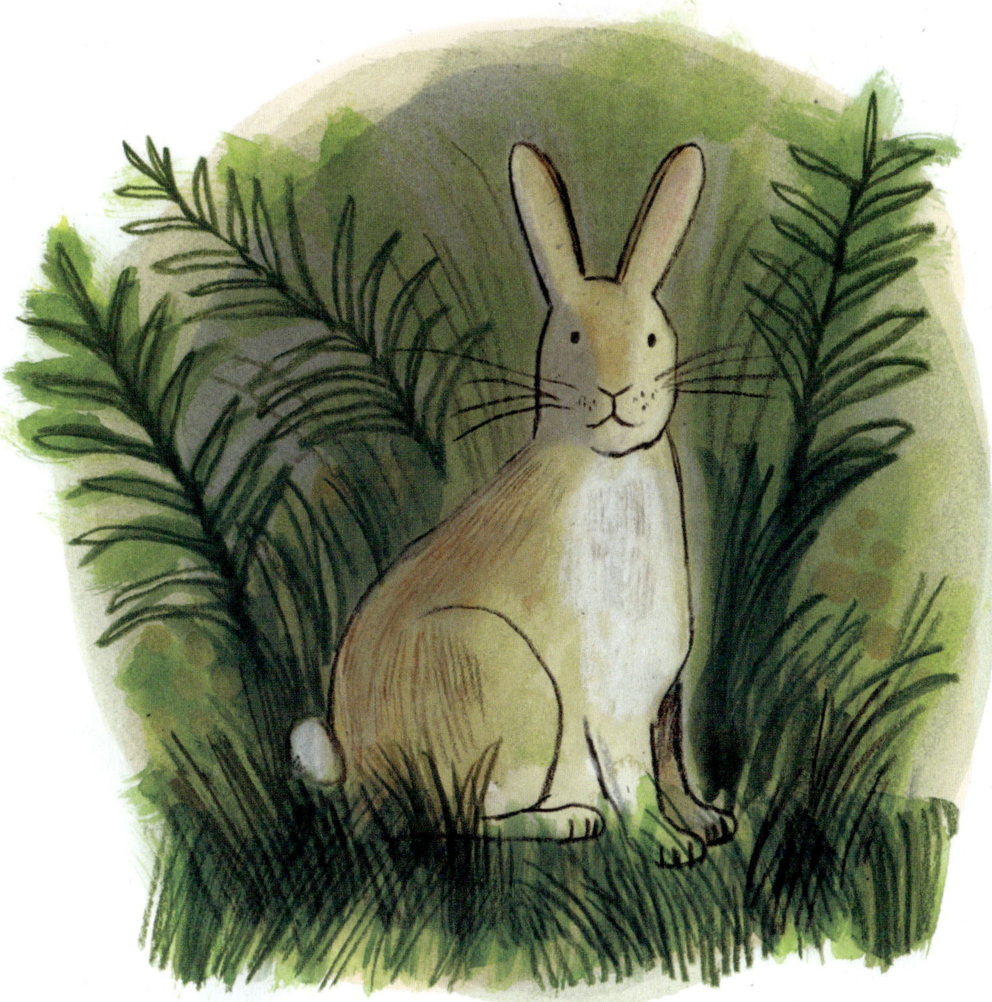

*When you love with your heart, there are no goodbyes.*

# The Velveteen Rabbit (or, How Toys Become Real)

## by Margery Williams

There was once a velveteen rabbit, and in the beginning he was really splendid. He was fat and bunchy, as a rabbit should be; his coat was spotted brown and white, he had real thread whiskers, and his ears were lined with pink sateen. On Christmas morning, when he sat wedged in the top of the Boy's stocking, with a sprig of holly between his paws, the effect was charming.

There were other things in the stocking, nuts and oranges and a toy engine, and chocolate almonds and a clockwork mouse, but the Rabbit was quite the best of all. For at least two hours the Boy loved him, and then Aunts and Uncles came to dinner, and there was a great rustling of tissue paper and unwrapping of parcels, and in the excitement of looking at all the new presents the Velveteen Rabbit was forgotten.

For a long time he lived in the toy cupboard or on the nursery floor, and no one thought very much about him. He was naturally shy, and being only made of velveteen, some of the more expensive toys quite snubbed him. The mechanical toys were very superior, and looked down upon everyone else; they were full of modern ideas, and pretended they were real. The model boat, who had lived through two seasons and lost most of his paint, caught the tone from them and never missed an opportunity of referring to his rigging in technical terms. The Rabbit could not claim to be a model of anything, for he didn't know that real rabbits existed; he thought they were all stuffed with sawdust like himself, and he understood that sawdust was quite out-of-date and should never be mentioned in modern circles. Even Timothy, the jointed wooden lion, who was made by the disabled soldiers, and should have had broader views, put on airs and pretended he was connected with Government. Between them all the poor little Rabbit was made to feel himself very insignificant and commonplace, and the only person who was kind to him at all was the Skin Horse.

The Skin Horse had lived longer in the nursery than any of the others. He was so old that his brown coat was bald in patches and showed the seams underneath, and most of the hairs in his tail had been pulled out to string bead necklaces. He was wise, for he had seen a long succession of mechanical toys arrive to boast and swagger, and by-and-by break their mainsprings and pass away, and he knew that they were only toys, and would never turn into anything else. For nursery magic is very strange and wonderful, and only those playthings that are old and wise and experienced like the Skin Horse understand all about it.

"What is REAL?" asked the Rabbit one day, when they were lying side by side near the nursery fender, before Nana came to tidy the room. "Does it mean having things that buzz inside you and a stick-out handle?"

"Real isn't how you are made," said the Skin Horse. "It's a thing that happens to you. When a child loves you for a long, long time, not just to play with, but REALLY loves you, then you become Real."

"Does it hurt?" asked the Rabbit.

"Sometimes," said the Skin Horse, for he was always truthful. "When you are Real you don't mind being hurt."

"Does it happen all at once, like being wound up," he asked, "or bit by bit?"

"It doesn't happen all at once," said the Skin Horse. "You become. It takes a long time. That's why it doesn't happen often to people who break easily, or have sharp edges, or who have to be carefully kept. Generally, by the time you are Real, most of your hair has been loved off, and your eyes drop out and you get loose in the joints and very shabby. But these things don't matter at all, because once you are Real you can't be ugly, except to people who don't understand."

"I suppose you are real?" said the Rabbit. And then he wished he had not said it, for he thought the Skin Horse might be sensitive. But the Skin Horse only smiled.

"The Boy's Uncle made me Real," he said. "That was a great many years ago; but once you are Real you can't become unreal again. It lasts for always."

The Rabbit sighed. He thought it would be a long time before this magic called Real happened to him. He longed to become Real, to know what it felt like; and yet the idea of growing shabby and losing his eyes and whiskers was rather sad. He wished that he could become it without these uncomfortable things happening to him.

There was a person called Nana who ruled the nursery. Sometimes she took no notice of the playthings lying about, and sometimes, for no reason whatever, she went swooping about like a great wind and hustled them away in cupboards. She called this "tidying up," and the playthings all hated it, especially the tin ones. The Rabbit didn't mind it so much, for wherever he was thrown he came down soft.

One evening, when the Boy was going to bed, he couldn't find the china dog that always slept with him. Nana was in a hurry, and it was too much trouble to hunt for china dogs at bedtime, so she simply looked about her, and seeing that the toy cupboard door stood open, she made a swoop.

"Here," she said, "take your old Bunny! He'll do to sleep with you!" And she dragged the Rabbit out by one ear, and put him into the Boy's arms.

That night, and for many nights after, the Velveteen Rabbit slept in the Boy's bed. At first he found it rather uncomfortable, for the Boy hugged him very tight, and sometimes he rolled over on him, and sometimes he pushed him so far under the pillow that the Rabbit could scarcely breathe. And he missed, too, those long moonlight hours in the nursery, when all the house was silent, and his talks with the Skin Horse. But very soon he grew to like it, for the Boy used to talk to him, and made nice tunnels for him under the bedclothes that he said were like the burrows the real rabbits lived in. And they had splendid games together, in whispers, when Nana had gone away to her supper and left the night-light burning on the mantelpiece. And when the Boy dropped off to sleep, the Rabbit would snuggle down close under his little warm chin and dream, with the Boy's hands clasped close round him all night long.

And so time went on, and the little Rabbit was very happy—so happy that he never noticed how his beautiful velveteen fur was getting shabbier and shabbier, and his tail becoming unsewn, and all the pink rubbed off his nose where the Boy had kissed him.

Spring came, and they had long days in the garden, for wherever the Boy went the Rabbit went too. He had rides in the wheelbarrow, and picnics on the grass, and lovely fairy huts built for him under the raspberry canes behind the flower border. And once, when the Boy was called away suddenly to go out to tea, the Rabbit was left out on the lawn until long after dusk, and Nana had to come and look for him with the candle because the Boy couldn't go to sleep unless he was there. He was wet through with the dew and quite earthy from diving into the burrows the Boy had made for him in the flower bed, and Nana grumbled as she rubbed him off with a corner of her apron.

"You must have your old Bunny!" she said. "Fancy all that fuss for a toy!"

The Boy sat up in bed and stretched out his hands.

"Give me my Bunny!" he said. "You mustn't say that. He isn't a toy. He's REAL!"

When the little Rabbit heard that he was happy, for he knew that what the Skin Horse had said was true at last. The nursery magic had happened to him, and he was a toy no longer. He was Real. The Boy himself had said it.

That night he was almost too happy to sleep, and so much love stirred in his little sawdust heart that it almost burst. And into his boot-button eyes, that had long ago lost their polish, there came a look of wisdom and beauty, so that even Nana noticed it next morning when she picked him up, and said, "I declare if that old Bunny hasn't got quite a knowing expression!"

That was a wonderful Summer!

Near the house where they lived there was a wood, and in the long June evenings the Boy liked to go there after tea to play. He took the Velveteen Rabbit with him, and before he wandered off to pick flowers, or play at brigands among the trees, he always made the Rabbit a little nest somewhere among the bracken, where he would be quite cosy, for he was a kind-hearted little boy and he liked Bunny to be comfortable. One evening, while the Rabbit was lying there alone, watching the ants that ran to and fro between his velvet paws in the grass, he saw two strange beings creep out of the tall bracken near him.

They were rabbits like himself, but quite furry and brand-new. They must have been very well made, for their seams didn't show at all, and they changed shape in a queer way when they moved; one minute they were long and thin and the next minute fat and bunchy, instead of always staying the same like he did. Their feet padded softly on the ground, and they crept quite close to him, twitching their noses, while the Rabbit stared hard to see which side the clockwork stuck out, for he knew that people who jump generally have something to wind them up. But he couldn't see it. They were evidently a new kind of rabbit altogether.

They stared at him, and the little Rabbit stared back. And all the time their noses twitched. "Why don't you get up and play with us?" one of them asked.

"I don't feel like it," said the Rabbit, for he didn't want to explain that he had no clockwork.

"Ho!" said the furry rabbit. "It's as easy as anything," And he gave a big hop sideways and stood on his hind legs.

"I don't believe you can!" he said.

"I can!" said the little Rabbit. "I can jump higher than anything!" He meant when the Boy threw him, but of course he didn't want to say so.

"Can you hop on your hind legs?" asked the furry rabbit.

That was a dreadful question, for the Velveteen Rabbit had no hind legs at all! The back of him was made all in one piece, like a pincushion. He sat still in the bracken, and hoped that the other rabbits wouldn't notice.

"I don't want to!" he said again.

But the wild rabbits have very sharp eyes. And this one stretched out his neck and looked.

"He hasn't got any hind legs!" he called out. "Fancy a rabbit without any hind legs!" And he began to laugh.

"I have!" cried the little Rabbit. "I have got hind legs! I am sitting on them!"

"Then stretch them out and show me, like this!" said the wild rabbit. And he began to whirl round and dance, till the little Rabbit got quite dizzy.

"I don't like dancing," he said. "I'd rather sit still!"

But all the while he was longing to dance, for a funny new tickly feeling ran through him, and he felt he would give anything in the world to be able to jump about like these rabbits did.

The strange rabbit stopped dancing, and came quite close. He came so close this time that his long whiskers brushed the Velveteen Rabbit's ear, and then he wrinkled his nose suddenly and flattened his ears and jumped backwards.

"He doesn't smell right!" he exclaimed. "He isn't a rabbit at all! He isn't real!"

"I am Real!" said the little Rabbit. "I am Real! The Boy said so!" And he nearly began to cry.

Just then there was a sound of footsteps, and the Boy ran past near them, and with a stamp of feet and a flash of white tails the two strange rabbits disappeared.

"Come back and play with me!" called the little Rabbit. "Oh, do come back! I know I am Real!"

But there was no answer, only the little ants ran to and fro, and the bracken swayed gently where the two strangers had passed. The Velveteen Rabbit was all alone.

"Oh, dear!" he thought. "Why did they run away like that? Why couldn't they stop and talk to me?"

For a long time he lay very still, watching the bracken, and hoping that they would come back. But they never returned, and presently the sun sank lower and the little white moths fluttered out, and the Boy came and carried him home.

Weeks passed, and the little Rabbit grew very old and shabby, but the Boy loved him just as much. He loved him so hard that he loved all his whiskers off, and the pink lining to his ears turned grey, and his brown spots faded. He even began to lose his shape, and he scarcely looked like a rabbit any more, except to the Boy. To him he was always beautiful, and that was all that the little Rabbit cared about. He didn't mind how he looked to other people, because the nursery magic had made him Real, and when you are Real, shabbiness doesn't matter.

And then, one day, the Boy was ill.

His face grew very flushed, and he talked in his sleep, and his little body was so hot that it burned the Rabbit when he held him close. Strange people came and went in the nursery, and a light burned all night and through it all the little Velveteen Rabbit lay there, hidden from sight under the bedclothes, and he never stirred, for he was afraid that if they found him some one might take him away, and he knew that the Boy needed him.

It was a long weary time, for the Boy was too ill to play, and the little Rabbit found it rather dull with nothing to do all day long. But he snuggled down patiently, and looked forward to the time when the Boy should be well again, and they would go out in the garden amongst the flowers and the butterflies and play splendid games in the raspberry thicket like they used to. All sorts of delightful things he planned, and while the Boy lay half asleep he crept up close to the pillow and whispered them in his ear. And presently the fever turned, and the Boy got better. He was able to sit up in bed and look at picture-books, while the little Rabbit cuddled close at his side. And one day, they let him get up and dress.

It was a bright, sunny morning, and the windows stood wide open. They had carried the Boy out on to the balcony, wrapped in a shawl, and the little Rabbit lay tangled up among the bedclothes, thinking.

The Boy was going to the seaside to-morrow. Everything was arranged, and now it only remained to carry out the doctor's orders. They talked about it all, while the little Rabbit lay under the bedclothes, with just his head peeping out, and listened. The room was to be disinfected, and all the books and toys that the Boy had played with in bed must be burnt.

"Hurrah!" thought the little Rabbit. "To-morrow we shall go to the seaside!" For the boy had often talked of the seaside, and he wanted very much to see the big waves coming in, and the tiny crabs, and the sand castles.

Just then Nana caught sight of him.

"How about his old Bunny?" she asked.

"That?" said the doctor. "Why, it's a mass of scarlet fever germs! Burn it at once. What? Nonsense! Get him a new one. He mustn't have that any more!"

And so the little Rabbit was put into a sack with the old picture-books and a lot of rubbish, and carried out to the end of the garden behind the fowl-house. That was a fine place to make a bonfire, only the gardener was too busy just then to attend to it. He had the potatoes to dig and the green peas to gather, but next morning he promised to come quite early and burn the whole lot.

That night the Boy slept in a different bedroom, and he had a new bunny to sleep with him. It was a splendid bunny, all white plush with real glass eyes, but the Boy was too excited to care very much about it. For to-morrow he was going to the seaside, and that in itself was such a wonderful thing that he could think of nothing else.

And while the Boy was asleep, dreaming of the seaside, the little Rabbit lay among the old picture-books in the corner behind the fowl-house, and he felt very lonely. The sack had been left untied, and so by wriggling a bit he was able to get his head through the opening and look out. He was shivering a little, for he had always been used to sleeping in a proper bed, and by this time his coat had worn so thin and threadbare from hugging that it was no longer any protection to him. Near by he could see the thicket of raspberry canes, growing tall and close like a tropical jungle, in whose shadow he had played with the Boy on bygone mornings. He thought of those long sunlit hours in the garden—how happy they were—and a great sadness came over him. He seemed to see them all pass before him, each more beautiful than the other, the fairy huts in the flower-bed, the quiet evenings in the wood when he lay in the bracken and the little ants ran over his paws; the wonderful day when he first knew that he was Real. He thought of the Skin Horse, so wise and gentle, and all that he had told him. Of what use was it to be loved and lose one's beauty and become Real if it all ended like this? And a tear, a real tear, trickled down his little shabby velvet nose and fell to the ground.

And then a strange thing happened. For where the tear had fallen a flower grew out of the ground, a mysterious flower, not at all like any that grew in the garden. It had slender green leaves the colour of emeralds, and in the centre of the leaves a blossom like a golden cup. It was so beautiful that the little Rabbit forgot to cry, and just lay there watching it. And presently the blossom opened, and out of it there stepped a fairy.

She was quite the loveliest fairy in the whole world. Her dress was of pearl and dew-drops, and there were flowers round her neck and in her hair, and her face was like the most perfect flower of all. And she came close to the little Rabbit and gathered him up in her arms and kissed him on his velveteen nose that was all damp from crying.

"Little Rabbit," she said, "don't you know who I am?"

The Rabbit looked up at her, and it seemed to him that he had seen her face before, but he couldn't think where.

"I am the nursery magic Fairy," she said. "I take care of all the playthings that the children have loved. When they are old and worn out and the children don't need them any more, then I come and take them away with me and turn them into Real."

"Wasn't I Real before?" asked the little Rabbit.

"You were Real to the Boy," the Fairy said, "because he loved you. Now you shall be Real to every one."

And she held the little Rabbit close in her arms and flew with him into the wood.

It was light now, for the moon had risen. All the forest was beautiful, and the fronds of the bracken shone like frosted silver. In the open glade between the tree-trunks the wild rabbits danced with their shadows on the velvet grass, but when they saw the Fairy they all stopped dancing and stood round in a ring to stare at her.

"I've brought you a new playfellow," the Fairy said. "You must be very kind to him and teach him all he needs to know in Rabbit-land, for he is going to live with you for ever and ever!"

And she kissed the little Rabbit again and put him down on the grass.

"Run and play, little Rabbit!" she said.

But the little Rabbit sat quite still for a moment and never moved. For when he saw all the wild rabbits dancing around him he suddenly remembered about his hind legs, and he didn't want them to see that he was made all in one piece. He did not know that when the Fairy kissed him that last time she had changed him altogether. And he might have sat there a long time, too shy to move, if just then something hadn't tickled his nose, and before he thought what he was doing he lifted his hind toe to scratch it.

And he found that he actually had hind legs! Instead of dingy velveteen he had brown fur, soft and shiny, his ears twitched by themselves, and his whiskers were so long that they brushed the grass. He gave one leap and the joy of using those hind legs was so great that he went springing about the turf on them, jumping sideways and whirling round as the others did, and he grew so excited that when at last he did stop to look for the Fairy she had gone.

He was a Real Rabbit at last, at home with the other rabbits.

Autumn passed and Winter, and in the Spring, when the days grew warm and sunny, the Boy went out to play in the wood behind the house. And while he was playing, two rabbits crept out from the bracken and peeped at him. One of them was brown all over, but the other had strange markings under his fur, as though long ago he had been spotted, and the spots still showed through. And about his little soft nose and his round black eyes there was something familiar, so that the Boy thought to himself:

"Why, he looks just like my old Bunny that was lost when I had scarlet fever!"

But he never knew that it really was his own Bunny, come back to look at the child who had first helped him to be Real.

## About the author

Harriet Griffey is a London-based journalist, writer, and internationally best-selling self-help author. She also teaches creative writing and facilitates writers' retreats. With a background in nursing, life coaching, and stress management, Harriet beautifully captures the universal truths and timeless themes of English-American author Margery Williams' classic text.

www.writersretreats.org

## About the illustrator

Harriet's words are brought vividly to life by Emma Carlisle—an award-nominated children's book illustrator, abstract painter, and landscape artist—whose stunning artwork thoughtfully reflects the beauty of the natural world.

Published in 2026 by
Rizzoli Universe, a division of
Rizzoli International Publications

Rizzoli International Publications Inc
49 West 27th Street
New York, NY 10001

Rizzoli International Publications UK Ltd
Somerset House, West Wing
Strand, London WC2R 1LA

www.rizzoliusa.com

Publisher: Charles Miers
Associate Publisher: Tina Persaud
Design: Kei Ishimaru
Production Manager: Michelle Wells
Reproduction: Rival UK
Senior Editor: Kristy Richardson



A CIP catalogue record for this book is available from the British Library.

ISBN: 9780789346773

MIX
Paper | Supporting responsible forestry
FSC® C005748
www.fsc.org

2026 / 1

Printed in China

The authorized representative in the EU for safety and compliance is Mondadori Libri S.p.A.,via Gian Battista Vico 42, Milan, Italy, 20123, www.mondadori.it

Visit us online: Instagram.com/RizzoliBooks
Facebook.com/RizzoliNewYork
Youtube.com/user/RizzoliNY